Health, Emotion and the Body

GILLIAN BENDELOW

polity

First published in 2009 by Polity Press

Polity Press
65 Bridge Street
Cambridge CB2 1UR, UK

Polity Press
350 Main Street
Malden, MA 02148, USA

ISBN-13: 978-0-7456-3643-6
ISBN-13: 978-0-7456-3644-3(paperback)

A catalogue record for this book is available from the British Library.

Typeset in 11 on 13pt Bembo
by SNP Best-set Typesetter Ltd., Hong Kong
Printed and bound in Great Britain by MPG Books Ltd, Bodmin, Cornwall

The publisher has used its best endeavours to ensure that the URLs for external websites referred to in this book are correct and active at the time of going to press. However, the publisher has no responsibility for the websites and can make no guarantee that a site will remain live or that the content is or will remain appropriate.

Every effort has been made to trace all copyright holders, but if any have been inadvertently overlooked the publishers will be pleased to include any necessary credits in any subsequent reprint or edition.

For further information on Polity, visit our website:
www.politybooks.com

Health, Emotion
and the Body

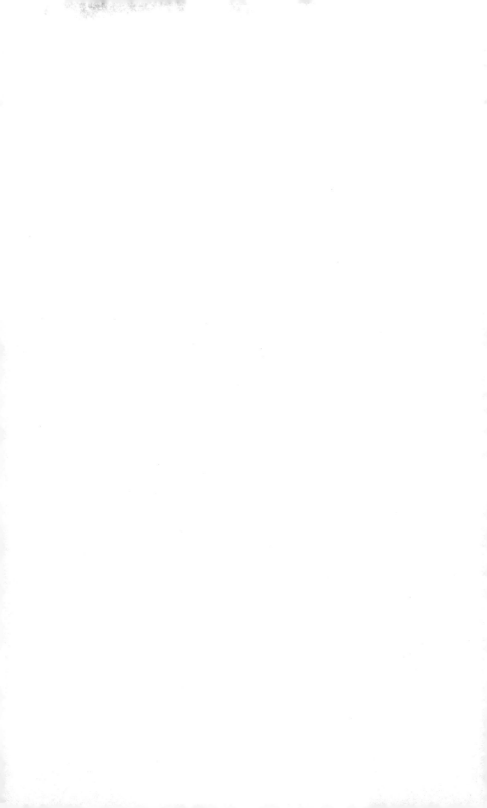

Contents

Preface

This book is concerned with understanding and explaining contemporary theories and models of health and illness, with regard to how they shape modern medical practice and healthcare, especially in relation to emotional, as well as physical, health. Central to this understanding is the critique of Cartesian dualism in scientific medicine, with its implicit separation of mind and body and creation of 'body machines'. Medical sociology has contributed a major challenge to the narrow philosophical grounding of biomedicine as illnesses of 'late modernity' feature multifactorial aetiologies and complex mind–body relationships which require traditional categories, formulations and management strategies to be re-evaluated; hence the turn to more holistic models of health and illness, which are now permeating medical education and practice.

In the light of these developments, more sophisticated conceptualizations of terms such as 'stress' and 'wellbeing' are needed to describe the intertwining of emotion and embodiment that occurs throughout the experience of health and illness. This book explores the limits of the division between 'mental' and 'physical' illnesses and charts these developments through a number of case study approaches within contemporary healthcare practice.

Chapter 1 begins by considering the range of explanations and associated conceptual models which describe the contemporary picture of health and illness in western society generally, and within the UK specifically. The conceptualization of stress is addressed in chapter 2, including recent work encapsulating social, as well as physiological and psychological, dimensions.

Chapter 3 examines medical categorizations of somatic disorders, in particular the phenomenon of *medically unexplained symptoms* (MUS) which is a source of extreme vexation and irritation to many physicians, and has resulted in the proliferation of a range of *contested conditions*. Chapter 4 explores the ever-expanding boundaries of the medicalization of emotional distress and 'dysfunction'. In turn, the highly publicized and controversial debates raging over our so-called *quick-fix culture*, invoked by encouragement of reliance on pharmaceutical and other medical solutions, address the thorny question of whether socially inappropriate behaviour can or should be seen as 'sickness'.

Chapter 5 addresses the increasing popularity of both complementary medicine and alternative healing systems, despite the focus on evidence-based medicine. Pluralistic healthcare practices have, of course, always existed within most societies, including those dominated by biomedicine, but the propensity to encompass mind/body divides and 'mop up' chronic limiting conditions such as back pain has been thought to have propelled the 'turn to holism' in an unprecedented manner during the latter half of the twentieth century.

Finally, the concluding chapter weighs up the benefits of a more integrated approach to healthcare, but also critically evaluates the more sinister surveillance implications and socially controlling aspects of 'healthism' in a society where individualism, consumerism and materialism are masked by emotional narcissism and the pursuit of bodily perfection.

Gillian Bendelow
October 2008

Acknowledgments

For Tess (again!)

Thanks to Ann Oakley, Jennie Popay and Berry Mayall for launching me on the academic path all those years ago, in the golden age of the origins of the Social Science Research Unit, and for being so inspirational.

Thanks to Paul Tyrrell, Vivien and Mario Cuccuru, and to my daughter Tess, who have constantly supported and encouraged me through all those years in every imaginable way.

Thanks to Colin Samson, Simon Williams and David Menkes for their collaboration in the study of emotion and embodiment, and to the many colleagues from the universities of Warwick and Sussex who have provided further inspiration.

Thanks to Sue Ziebland for giving me permission to use the quotations from DipEx interviews (now renamed Health Talkonline), and to the friends and family (some of whom are no longer with us) whose poignant stories have helped to illustrate how distress is acted out so powerfully through our minds and bodies.

Gillian Bendelow

1
Beyond Biomedicalization: Integrated Models of Health and Illness

Key concepts: biomedical/social/integrated models; evidence-based medicine; values-based medicine; medicalization; mind/body dualism

In the early twenty-first century, health and illness are multi-faceted concepts which span a range of disciplines and have varied meanings across cultures and societies (Helman 2007; Blaxter 2004). Since the nineteenth century we have witnessed dramatic advances in the understanding and cure of disease with, at least in so-called 'western' or 'developed' countries, an unprecedented extension of both quality and length of life (in this book, 'western medicine' signifies health-care practice and organization which shares general characteristics across Northern and Western Europe, Scandinavia, Northern America and Australasia).

Yet even as medical science has progressed, there has been an equally dramatic decline of faith, exacerbated in recent years by a series of scandals – in the UK over the last decade, for instance, there has been a continuous stream of media stories of 'dirty hospitals', removal of organs without consent, and doctors who may be serial killers at worst or negligent at best. The dominance and certainty of biomedicine has been challenged by litigation, scandal, government regulation, lay expertise and social activism (Fox 2002; Scambler 2004) and continues to face increasing controversy and challenge in the new millennium. Traditionally, medical sociologists have posited a distinction between disease and illness (Dingwall 1976; Helman 2007) to convey a polarization between the natural world of biological processes and social responses to disease; and to some extent, this book attempts to elaborate this position, but is particularly concerned with charting more recent attempts to provide *integrated* or *holistic* accounts of contemporary healthcare.

Models of health, illness and disease

Theories about the *aetiology* of disease and illness may rely heavily on one particular orientation, or they may be multi-causal. For example, explanations which favour lifestyle explanations obviously point to social factors, but are also under the control of individual choices about healthy/non-healthy behaviour. Table 1.1 demonstrates how differing factors may provide a single overarching theory (as in some accounts of germ theory or environmental factors) or may combine several perspectives (the larger the 'X' the more significant the explanation).

Thus, these theoretical frameworks can be dynamic, and are not necessarily fixed, but their authority and implementation in mainstream healthcare provision relies on research evidence which inevitably is validated by the scientific medical community. Consequently, the biomedical model and evidence-based medicine are, and are likely to remain, the most dominant and powerful models in the healthcare

Table 1.1   Aetiologies of illness and disease

Type of explanation	Biological	Social	Psychological/ emotional
Germ theory	X		
Genetic	X	x	
Immunity	X	x	x
Environmental		X	
Lifestyle		x	X

approaches described in this book, even though that authority is increasingly under challenge.

The biomedical model

The term *medical model* is used interchangeably to mean both a sociological 'ideal type' constructed to differentiate an orientation towards disease that reflects dominant medical theory, and 'the pre-eminent scientific model used by those involved with medical science for the explanation of disease'; it is also known as the *biomedical model* (Hansen and Easthope 2006).

The development of a biologically deterministic model of health and illness is historically linked with the rise of the medical profession. 'Medicalization', in turn, is a strand in the nature/nurture debate which has a long history, centred on the interaction between biological and cultural determinism.

Historians of medicine show that the notion of 'disease' can be traced back to Hippocrates, with the postulation that a combination of signs and symptoms can be observed to occur together so frequently and so characteristically as to constitute a recognizable and typical clinical picture, a model highly influenced by the philosophy of René Descartes in the seventeenth century. Descartes saw the mind as activating the will of the human spirit through the subordinate physical matter of the body, a view in opposition to the predominant philosophical stance of orthodox Christianity on the inseparability of body and soul. This enforced inseparability had until then retarded the development of medical science by forbidding dissection; as well as these revolutionary implications for anatomical study, the philosophical reflections of Descartes did, of course, have a profound influence on the development of positivist science. Logical thought based on empirical observation was emphasized, laying the foundations of the mechanistic biomedical approach which is so characteristic of medicine, or rather what is termed 'western medicine' or 'modern medicine'.

'Western biomedicine' has often been characterized as the scientific system of medicine which superseded earlier 'magical' or religious ways of dealing with health and illness as part of the much wider shift to rationality associated with the Enlightenment linked to processes of industrialization, urbanization, liberal democracy and the 'march of progress' of modernity in all walks of life as well as in science. The claims of the Enlightenment reflect the ideology of the inexorable march of medical progress, with the 'battle against disease' being won and influenced by the earlier work of Thomas Sydenham (1624–89), known as 'the English Hippocrates', who emphasized the need to differentiate illnesses from each other. A doctrine was generated by the work of Louis Pasteur (1822–95), and of Robert Koch (1843–1910), who demonstrated that disease has specific causes which can be identified and treated. The separate and specific aetiologies of infectious diseases such as scarlet fever, measles, gout, smallpox and malaria were thus identified, and germ theory has dominated 'western' medicine since the nineteenth century.

Implicit in this model are the following notions:

- that health is a natural and desired state of nature
- that health is the absence of diagnosable disease
- that identifiable diseases have specific biological causes combated by specific counter remedies.

Even within biological models of illness aetiology there are competing explanations. For example, there are theories about immunity in which the body is invaded by external pathogens but does not necessarily succumb and may either win or lose the fight (Martin 1994). More controversially, genetic explanations focus on mutations which can act to predispose to illness as in breast cancer and coronary heart disease, or to result in single gene disorders such depression and alcoholism. Other major features of the biomedical model include an orientation towards *cure*, towards the manipulation of organic symptoms with the intention of effecting their disappearance; the perception of *disease* as an autonomous and potentially manageable entity which threatens personal health in a temporary or episodic fashion; a focus on the isolated *individual* as the site of the disease and the appropriate object of treatment, and a belief that the most appropriate place for treatment is a *medical environment* – the consulting room or the hospital – not the environment where symptoms arise. Parsons' influential theory (1951) of the sick role underpins many of the assumptions of biomedicine, including the polarization of illness and health and the unquestioning normalization of the patient cooperating with the doctor to be well again and that prevention is an individual responsibility to avoid risk. The emphasis on specific disease categories resulted in the body being considered analogous to a machine (hence the profusion of 'engineering' metaphors), whose individual parts could be examined and treated without the rest of the body being affected, serving to deflect attention away from the environment and the individual's relationship to it. Again, without question, doctors are the trained experts who understand objectively the workings of the body, know how to correct problems by technological interventions, often in high-technology hospitals surrounding the social relations of high-technology medicine.

The biomedical paradigm, which has dominated medicine throughout the twentieth century and onwards, gains much of its credibility from the association of scientific breakthroughs with dramatic declines in mortality rates. Use of the biomedical model for research on health and illness has resulted in a focus on the production and analysis of statistics of mortality and morbidity. Medical, and to a large extent social, research in the health field has traditionally been dominated by positivism and by an alignment with the medico-scientific method. It can also be linked to the critique of rationality in which health and illness no longer have any intrinsic meaning such as punishment from God for man's ills. Instead, human beings' physical selves are subject to the laws of nature. During the twentieth century the rationalization process was accelerated by the prolific growth and development of evidence-based medicine.

Evidence-based medicine

Although the testing of medical interventions for efficacy can be traced back for centuries, during the twentieth century this practice evolved as a paradigm which has impacted hugely on all forms of medical practice and healthcare policy. In 1972 Archie Cochrane, an epidemiologist, published *Effectiveness and Efficiency: Random Reflections on Health Services,* which sparked a whole movement in evidence-based medicine (EBM), the process of applying the scientific method to medical practice. This led to the development of the Cochrane collaboration and the Cochrane Centres within the UK. The term evidence-based medicine entered common parlance in medical literature in the early 1990s and has become internationally dominant, defined as 'the conscientious, explicit and judicious use of current best evidence in making decisions about the care of individual patients' by the Oxford Centre for Evidence-Based Medicine (www.cebm. net).

The aims of EBM are to ensure individual patients are treated in accordance with the most scientifically valid findings, and that in turn these findings are under a systematic process of continual evaluation and comparison to ensure best practice. In this model the 'gold standard' of research is held up as the randomized, double-blind, placebo-controlled trial which is regarded as being bias- and value-free. The practice of EBM has an implicit agenda of clinical expertise, not only in being able to diagnose and treat illness, but also in being seen as actively involved in good practice, able to interpret and evaluate clinical findings, and able to communicate the risks and benefits of these effectively to patients as well as to other clinicians, academic forums and the general public.

Whilst these aims and principles are to be admired and upheld, EBM has also been accused of reductionism, in common with other criticisms of the biomedical model, in that all dysfunction can be attributed to causal biochemical changes, and of exclusionary properties as alternative perspectives are rendered invalid (Tonelli 1998). For example, there is a tendency in EBM to prioritize the biological germ theory based on single causation, in contrast to other multicausal theories of disease, for example those based on immunity, genetics, environment and lifestyle (see table 1.1). Furthermore, in this model patients' testimonies and experience of illness are seen as subjective and unreliable, and are disregarded as sources of data. As with the biomedical model more generally, complete reliance on EBM in medical research has been charged with providing an incomplete picture of contemporary patterning of health and illness.

The 'crisis' and critique of biomedicine

Over the course of the twentieth century, in Britain, the United States and Western Europe the major killers, infectious diseases, were largely replaced by degenerative illnesses such as coronary heart disease and cancer, illnesses with multicausal aetiologies and complex mind–body relationships. Sontag's famous metaphorical analysis of biomedicine as military manoeuvre gained momentum (Sontag 1978) but the claims of 'victory' in the 'battle' against disease were, to some extent, undermined in the latter half of the twentieth century by clinical uncertainty and public distrust. These phenomena were, in turn, fuelled by social movements such as feminism, anti-racism and the disability movement, and by political economists of health who highlighted the divide between rich and poor in access and resources to medicine. The profession was accused of 'elitism' in stark contrast to the heroic claims of the 'golden age' at the beginning of the nineteenth century, when the metaphors of waging war and battling against disease became reality with the discovery of 'magic bullets' to eradicate most of the major infectious killers and the amazing increase in life expectancy, at least in the 'western' world.

As medical sociology, with its largely functionalist beginnings, began to transform into the sociology of health and illness, the 'radical critique' drew heavily on the work of Foucault to begin to address how the rise of biomedicine could be shown to be socially and historically constructed as both a system of scientific knowledge and a paradigm of the social organization of health and illness (Armstrong 1983; Petersen and Bunton 1997). Foucault's 'political anatomy' is based on mechanisms of power rather than progressive enlightenment or random effect; his 'clinical gaze' demonstrates how changing ideologies of disease can be seen as a product of differing perceptions of the body:

> Disease is no longer a bundle of characters dissociated here and there over the surface of a body and linked together by statistically observable concomitances and successions; it is a set of forms and deformations, figures and accidents, and of displaced, destroyed or modified elements bound together in sequence according to a geography which can be followed step by step. It is no longer a pathological species inserting itself into the body whenever possible; it is the body itself which becomes ill. (Foucault 1973: 136)

From the late nineteenth century, as Jewson (1974) so vividly depicted, the rise of scientific medicine resulted in the shift of focus from the whole person to the disease located in the biological cell (literally from the bedside to the hospital and then to the laboratory). Just as the biomedical model rose, so it has the potential to fall, and many claim we are living in a period where such a fall or diminution in its power is occurring.

Many writers have discussed the concept of *medical uncertainty* in this phenomenon, and have drawn attention to the dilemmas which arise from the tension between the particular and the general in healthcare practice. Fox (2002) has helpfully analysed these tensions on different levels.

First she points to the *epistemological uncertainty* faced by health professionals when using medicial evidence generated through studies of populations, such as clinical trials and epidemiology, and applying this evidence to individual patients. For example, we know that smoking is a likely cause of cancer but a doctor does not know if the patient sitting in front of them will get cancer or not. Second, there is uncertainty because of a lack of a conceptual framework for our understanding. For example, how can the new knowledge about the human genome (our genetic make-up) be combined with knowledge about other biological and social dimensions of medicine and health to be of use to the practice of medicine? Medicine does not have a conceptual framework for linking up the different levels of understanding related to health from genes through physiology, psychology, family, community and society.

Finally, there is uncertainty about the balance between the individual and distributive ethic of medicine. For example, what is the appropriate balance between attending to individuals' health needs and attending to the health needs of a population, and what benefits and disbenefits does attending to the one have for the other? For example, attending to population health needs may cause disruption for some individuals. Likewise, attending to individual needs may use resources that could have been used for the needs of the population.

The proliferation of ethical concerns and dilemmas is addressed in the development of values-based medicine.

Values-based medicine

Values-based medicine (VBM) has developed from within medical practice (Fulford, Dickenson and Murray 2002) with the tacit principle that healthcare delivery and treatment can never be a purely scientific enterprise. Human beings, whether delivering or receiving healthcare, are fundamentally subjective and value-laden beings. Some areas of medical practice, such as primary care and psychiatry in particular, are intrinsically value-laden, and rather than being in opposition to and arguing against evidence-based medicine, as is often assumed, VBM offers a framework to conduct a process of 'ethical reasoning' to ensure good practice. VBM builds on interdisciplinary and humanistic principles of open communication, mutual respect and emotional connection between physicians and their patients, termed 'relationship-centred' or 'patient-centred' care in contrast to 'disease-centred' care, and accepts that subjective experiences are important aspects of diagnosis and treatment.

Although VBM accepts the four basic principles of bioethics, namely autonomy, beneficence, non-maleficence and justice (Beauchamp and Childress 1994), the process of ethical reasoning differs radically from the quasi-legal and prescriptive bioethical guidelines. Fulford et al. claim that this approach may be more abstract theoretically (ergo less rigid) but it is also concrete because it relies on the results of empirical studies (Fulford et al. 2002: 9).

Values-based medicine feeds into the development of integrated models, as it highlights the role of communication skills, the relationship between ethics and law, and the role of medical humanities in medical practice. Methodologically, it provides an enormous challenge to the dominance of positivism, and the last decade has seen an unprecedented acceptance of qualitative studies published in medical journals, with conceptual frameworks of such illness experience and narrative medicine becoming mainstream in medical research and teaching practice, rather than confined to social science and literature. VBM also allows for a fundamentally interdisciplinary approach, linking science to social science and humanities, and emphasizes the importance of social models in understanding and explaining health and illness.

Social models

A major critique of biomedicine came from within the profession when McKeown (1979) used large-scale analyses of available epidemiological statistics of mortality decline in England and Wales to argue that the contribution of medical intervention had been overemphasized, and that most of the decline in mortality from infectious disease occurred before effective immunization became available, with the possible exception of smallpox and diphtheria. McKeown's thesis restates the main determinants of the public health as improvements in environmental health measures leading to better sanitation and a purer water supply, plus limitations in family size and, most importantly, improved nutrition. This was backed up by further research from Szreter (1988), emphasizing that the role of nutrition in this debate was important as social factors became an issue, with the focus on social and external factors such as diet, housing, pollution and sanitation. There was also an implicit association with industrialization and socioeconomic inequality politicized through activism; in other words, disease can be seen as a direct result of government policy and capitalist greed.

A plethora of sociological critiques of the biomedical model have contributed to a widespread recognition of the limitations of biomedicine and to the development of more holistic and integrated approaches to practice, teaching and research (Wade and Halligan 2004). Social sciences associated with medicine, particularly medical sociology, philosophy/bioethics and health psychology, have shaped modern ideas about health and illness and over the course of the twentieth century formed a major challenge to the somewhat narrow philosophical grounding of biomedicine. Since the second half of the twentieth century, important influences include:

- critiques from within social movements (social class, gender, ethnicity, sexuality and disability)
- sophisticated social theories of emotion, embodiment, illness and disability
- the growth of lay knowledge and user movements
- regulation and professionalization
- public understandings of science and knowledge especially through new information technology
- the popularity of complementary and alternative medicine
- medicalization and healthism critiques.

In order to analyse the social status and context of health and illness in contemporary 'western society', this book draws on these critiques to underpin the topics outlined in the preface, and, in particular, attempts to link understandings of the medicalization process to our emotionally expressive bodies.

Medicalization and 'body machines'

The medicalization thesis emerged in the mid twentieth century with social commentators such as Illich (1975) and Zola (1972) expressing concern at the process whereby, throughout the twentieth century, medicine became annexed to areas of so-called 'ordinary' life which may have been previously under moral, religious or legal jurisdiction. As well as birth and death, which had traditionally taken place in the home in past ages, this phenomenon has been extended in the twenty-first century to all aspects of human reproduction (including menstruation, childbirth, abortion, contraception, reproductive technology and menopause), as well as the regulation of emotional behaviour through psychiatry and psychosocial interventions into behavioural dysfunction including substance misuse. More recently our very identity and appearance have become medicalized through body weight regulation, beauty treatments and cosmetic surgery (Black 2004). Thus a whole range of behaviours and conditions are given medical meanings and defined in terms of health and illness, even though some critics claim this is inappropriate (see chapter 3).

Strong (1977) coined the term medical *imperialism* to imply how medicine as an institution of social control eliminates or controls problematic experiences defined as deviant in order to enforce adherence to social norms. On an ideological level this process destroys traditional resources and creates dependence and passivity in patients (Illich 1975). Medicalization is both *conceptual* in that medical vocabulary is used to define a problem and *institutional* in that the problem is legitimated when diagnosis and/or treatment occurs (Reissman 1989).

Whilst the advancement of medical knowledge undoubtedly benefited enormously from the profound insights of Descartes, it has also been argued that the Cartesian 'revolution' has severely limited the scope of western medicine as ancient theoretical dichotomies, rooted in ancient Greek philosophy, were given added weight by Descartes, who:

> at the beginning of the modern era, argued persuasively that the only path to knowledge was the scientific side of the dichotomy and that we must ignore or control the artistic side. This one-sided mechanistic view was applied to medicine, and the body and disease processes came to be seen in those terms.
> (Wagner 1982: 1207)

Anti-dualist philosophers such as Ryle (1949) further emphasized the dangers and limitations of proposing two collateral but separate histories of the mind and of the body, resulting in a strenuous campaign against Cartesian dualism threading through postmodern and feminist writings in particular.

Although it is important to make the distinction between Descartes' original work and the way in which medicine may have crudely appropriated aspects of his theory, the reductionism of the mind–body split has become one of the most heavily criticized features of the biomedical model. A powerful example of the dangers of this crude reductionism can be seen in the second-wave feminist critiques of the medicalization of reproduction. Human reproduction is one of the most significant sites for the meeting of both biological and social meanings and histories, and claims that discourses of medicine as agent of social control combined with the social construction of gender and sexuality within medicine have 'historically constituted a site of sexual discrimination using medico-scientific justifications for differentiating between men and women on the basis of "biology" and anatomy' (Martin 1987: 17). Although medicalized childbirth has undoubtedly brought enormous benefits in release from pain, infection and death, the technologized birth, in the form of monitoring, forceps, artificial induction, anaesthesia, episiotomy and caesarean sections, also came under scrutiny and criticism, with women's experience being sidelined for medical goals of healthy babies in which the 'normal' birth is a social construction rather than a biological fact (Oakley 1984).

Many feminists claim that dominant societal definitions of women as reproducers mean that health professionals see their bodies as mere machines, which are inherently defective and in need of medical intervention, as in this much-cited classic quote from an eminent North American gynaecologist, Dr Waldo Fielding:

> The female anatomy is not made to have babies – she was designed to be a four-legged animal. Instead she stands on two feet, so the entire weight of pregnancy doesn't hang free, but sits on large vessels, causing fluid to build up in extremities . . . furthermore there isn't a cervix owned by any woman that doesn't tear. (*The Boston Globe* in 1894: quoted in Oakley 1984)

Whereas the traditional feminist critiques of the 1970s and 1980s picked up on the notion of medicine as 'imperialist', perpetrating iatrogenic interventions on passive women 'victims', feminism itself came under fire with assertions that women were not a homogeneous group, and that some women were 'more equal than others'. On the one hand socially controlling reproductive technologies such as enforced contraception and abortions may be aimed at socially 'undesirable' women, whereas on the other hand some affluent and highly educated women seek out and demand interventions such as cosmetic surgery and caesarean section. Revisionist accounts point to the benefits of medicalization for women's lives, and the freedoms we have experienced since the twentieth century, pointing out that women have always been active if not equal participants in the process, and thus have both gained and lost (Reissman 1989). Furthermore, the pathologization of women's bodies is not the sole creation of medical practices; nevertheless clinical encounters reflect and reinforce prevailing views in society. Sociologists of emotion have highlighted how emotions provide the link between mind and body, nature and culture, structure and action, and are able to transcend some of the dichotomous ways of thinking which act to limit social thought and investigation, including the division between masculine and feminine (Hochschild 1983; Bendelow and Williams 1998). In turn, the consequences of Cartesian dualism have become a central issue, particularly in work on the body (Bordo and Jagger 1987; Grosz 1994), on the social control of medicine over women's reproductive lives (Oakley 1984; Martin 1987), and within the wider epistemological critiques of science and knowledge (see for example Smith 1988; Haraway 1991; Rose 1994). These critiques challenge the powerfully dominant model, which sees the 'natural' in terms of bodies and emotions as essentially female and thus inferior to male 'rationality', and argue for a more unified 'feminine' conception of reason which accepts emotions and sexuality as having an important role in the acquisition of knowledge.

Doctor–patient relationships have transformed from the functional consensual model of the sick role, characterized by obedience and unquestioning acceptance of clinical expertise, to negotiated models of interaction between healthcare professionals and the lay population. New forms of technology, the Internet in particular, mean that unprecedented levels and exchange of information inform the lay–expert interaction and subsequent participation in the medicalization process. Recent debates have contended that indeed recipients of healthcare are not merely passive recipients of health technologies but may see themselves more as consumers. Moreover, clinicians themselves have criticized the tendency for the general public to turn to medicine to 'cure' inappropriate afflictions of everyday life, as indicated by table 1.2 which demonstrates the least popular consultations experienced by general practitioners in a poll conducted by the *British Medical Journal*.

Despite the advances of modern medicine, healthcare systems in wealthy countries including the UK are facing enormous difficulties in meeting demand, distributing resources and providing adequate care. As these healthcare systems become larger and more bureaucratic, both practitioners and patients experience dehumanization.

Table 1.2   Top 20 non-diseases in descending order

1. Ageing
2. Work
3. Boredom
4. Bags under eyes
5. Ignorance
6. Baldness
7. Freckles
8. Big ears
9. Grey or white hair
10. Ugliness
11. Childbirth
12. Allergy to 21st century
13. Jet lag
14. Unhappiness
15. Cellulite
16. Hangover
17. Anxiety about penis size
18. Pregnancy
19. Road rage
20. Loneliness

Source: R. Smith (2002)

Dissatisfaction and disillusionment with biomedicine is endemic, in particular the depersonalization and fragmentation experienced through the perceived effects of Cartesian dualism and the 'body as machine' model which has permeated western scientific medicine. Poor doctor–patient relationships result in lawsuits against healthcare providers and, for practitioners, the fear of litigation plus high levels of stress and burnout mean they are often unable to give individual patients the attention they need. Added to the dismantling of welfarism and the rising cost of medical services, the two-tier system of private insurance versus the National Health Service means that many receive inadequate healthcare.

Paradoxically, as the lay voice has become more widely heard through consumerism and other challenges to medical power, the popularity of therapies and treatments which integrate mind and body has grown in a 'turn to holism' among the population who can pay for healthcare.

The turn towards holism

The rise of biomedicine has been linked with a tendency for western industrialized societies to live in relative isolation from natural forces and even to remain somewhat impervious to seasonal shifts. Living in harmony and in direct experiential connection with the natural world loses its centrality in modern life and shifts in social and medical worldviews away from holism and towards atomization are normalized.

Before the dominance of the biomedical paradigm, the elements of earth, air, fire and water were linked to the humours of the body. Engels (1987 [1845]) linked health to the environment in his descriptions of industrializing London when arguing that 'bad air' (pollution) in slums caused by the social and economic activities of industrialization were the cause of widespread morbidity and mortality in working-class people – a phenomenon tantamount to social murder. Helman's (2007) exposition of lay conceptions of everyday maladies such as colds and fevers indicates that while people draw on germ theory to make sense of what causes their cold or fever, they also speak in terms of harmony with their natural surroundings and of bodily humours – linkages exemplified in their explanations that catching a chill caused them to catch a cold (see also Blaxter 2004: 32–3). Furthermore, Blaxter (2004) cites miasma as an example of a disease caused by climate, while Dubos (1987) suggests that the modern concept of fitness (the ability of the organism to resist the impact of the outside world and maintain homeostasis in the internal environment) links the Hippocratic dictum that health is universal sympathy with the modern conception of immunity (see Martin 1994).

By the 1980s, propelled by the 'cultural critique', the 'new' public health, lay knowledge and user movements, managerialism, litigation and the professionalization of nursing further undermined medical power. The rise in popularity of holistic, alternative and complementary therapies in contemporary society at this point in time can be linked in particular to the criticism of Cartesian dualism and the body–mind reductionism of biomedical approaches. The following extracts from two medical textbooks both published in the 1970s, one British, one translated from Chinese, vividly illustrate the conceptual difference between biomedical and holistic models of health and illness in healthcare practice.

Comparative texts

In a traditional medical textbook for nurses in its 12th edition (Bloom 1979), the heading of aetiology typically portrays a somewhat restricted conception of the causes of disease as follows (1979: 8–9):

> The term aetiology is used to denote causation of disease. There are thousands of possible causes and the following classification gives only the main ones:
>
> 1. *Living organisms or microbes*
>   a) Bacteria
>   b) Viruses
>   c) Fungi
>   d) Parasites
> 2. *Physical and chemical agents*
>   a) Injury (trauma)
>   b) Excesses of heat or cold

    c)   Electricity, X-rays and radioactive substances
    d)   Toxic drugs
    e)   Poisonous gases
    f)   Cigarette smoking
3. *Deficiency and hormonal diseases*
    Lack or disturbance of:
    a)   Vitamins
    b)   Hormones
    c)   Diet
4. *Heredity*
5. *Autoimmune diseases*
6. *Unknown* (including causes of tumours)

In contrast, the following extract from *A Barefoot Doctor's Manual* (Revolutionary Health Committee of Hunan Province 1978) demonstrates how, in Chinese traditional medicine, emotional and external factors are intrinsic to understanding the causes of illness and disease. This section concerning the causes of disease begins in a similar manner by discussing signs, symptoms and physical examination results as the first step in the diagnosis of the disease. However, in order to make a correct diagnosis, the practitioner:

> must make an overall study of the patient's attitudes, mental activity and illness to correctly differentiate between the aetiology and the present course of the disease. The human body is an integral mechanism in which inconsistencies contradict each other. It also has a very close relationship with society and its natural environment. The onset and development of disease frequently are related to the body's makeup, its resistance and the virulence and number of pathogens present, in a complex relationship. (1978: 25)

The manual then describes causal factors related to individual physiological dispositions under the heading of *body factors*, but in this account, emotional activity is intrinsic to the process:

BODY FACTORS

1. *Nervous and emotional make-up:* Mental and emotional activity among different individuals vary under the

different influences of society and the natural environment. Examples are joy, excitement, happiness, anger, fright and sorrow. Under most conditions, emotional activity will not cause disease, but under certain conditions it can damage normal body function and cause or hasten its development, e.g. certain neuroses or functional digestive disturbances. However, we must feel the dynamic effect of the proletarian world view and its revolutionary optimism on preventing or overwhelming disease. For example, some of our comrades who have incurred serious burns, because they can hold on to a fearless revolutionary determination to fight against disease, ultimately overcome it. This fully explains the dynamic the patient's subjective outlook can have on overcoming a serious illness.

2. *Body make-up or physical conditions:* This includes the body build, body reactions and differences such as age, sex, resistance to disease, which are closely related to the incurrence and development of disease. After 1950, the large working masses were given regular training so their bodies may become healthy and strong, and less susceptible to disease. Furthermore, the aged or the young, because of a weak body make-up, may, because of weak resistance, be easily affected by disease-causing factors to become ill. The human body's reactions to external environmental and internal body factors may vary because of regional, age, sex and sensitivity differences. For example, children can easily be affected by infantile paralysis, while older adults are more susceptible to cancer. Some people are allergic to pollen, shrimp and crab, and develop wheezing or urticaria. Certain other ailments are commonly seen in men, and others more commonly seen in females. These are all closely related to the human body's reaction.

The manual then moves on to take a much broader approach under the heading of *external factors*, taking into account a wide range of social and environmental factors, thus:

EXTERNAL FACTORS: These include various social and natural environmental factors. Sometimes etiologic factors are quite complex.

Social factors: Differences in the social system often have a great effect on the incidence and elimination of certain diseases. China has early eliminated cholera, smallpox, venereal disease, plague, etc. With respect to certain diseases with more serious consequences such as malaria and schistosomiasis, better prevention and treatment measures have greatly reduced the disease incidence. Therefore, when causes of disease are analysed, great emphasis must be given to the social system.

Physical factors: e.g. Radiation, mechanical injuries, war injuries, high altitude, high temperature, outer space activity, etc.

Chemical factors: e.g. Strong acids and alkalis, pharmaceuticals, cyanide products, organic phosphorus in agricultural insecticides, and snake venom.

Biological factors: e.g. Pathogenic viruses, bacteria, fungi, spirochetes, protozoa, tapeworms, etc. Biological pathogens attacking the human body are quite selective in their site of attack.

Climactic factors: Under normal conditions, natural climatic factors, such as wind, cold, heat, humidity, aridity, etc. do not cause disease but if the climate changes suddenly and the body's resistance is lowered and cannot adapt immediately, the above elements are linked to certain symptoms in traditional Chinese medicine.

Other factors: e.g. Unhygienic eating habits that lack discipline and control can also be indirect pathological factors.
(Revolutionary Health Committee of Hunan Province 1978: 25–6)

The extract demonstrates a fundamentally holistic approach to illness, in stark contrast to the mechanistic, dualist biomedical model which is unable systematically to take on board the aetiological role.

Traditional and alternative healing systems

Folk medicine, herbal remedies and 'lay' healing practices have existed since antiquity, and alternative healing systems have continued to proliferate even then the advent of biomedicine (often termed scientific, allopathic or 'western' medicine). Many writers claim that the myriad of healthcare systems and practices of complementary and alternative medicines (known collectively by conventional medicine as CAM, a somewhat problematic acronym which will be discussed more fully in chapter 5) have always existed alongside allopathic medicine. The practices referred to by the acronym CAM currently subsume the following broad categories:

• Psychological treatment and support (psychotherapy, imagery, group therapy, cancer support groups)
• Nutritional approaches and herbal remedies
• Massage and relaxation techniques
• Psychic healing (prayer, laying on of hands)
• Alternative healing systems (Ayurvedism, traditional Chinese medicine (TCM), homeopathy, naturopathy).

The lumping together of so many different and, indeed, paradoxical categories under the CAM rubric makes it a highly problematic working concept. Pietroni (1992) once jibed that to speak of alternative medicine was like the English talking about 'foreigners' – both terms were vaguely pejorative, referring to large heterogeneous categories defined by what they are not rather than by what they are.

For a variety of cultural, social, economic or scientific reasons, CAM has been largely excluded by conventional biomedicine. Although some specialist areas (e.g. pain clinics, oncology, liaison psychiatry) are developing integrated theory and practice, it is still much the case that conventional 'western' healthcare professionals remain ill prepared to usefully understand and apply the connections between mental and physical health. By contrast, an integrated mind–body concept is central to most forms of complementary or alternative medicine and the idea of fundamental energies flowing in and through the body is explicit in most 'alternative' philosophies about health and healing. Indeed, an emphasis on notions of balance and energy links the more widely accepted therapies such as homeopathy, acupuncture and naturopathy with those more easily dismissed as 'fringe' medicine such as traditional Hindu (Ayurvedic) and Chinese medicine. Given this view, the disruption of energies and energy pathways in the body, their blocking and the resultant 'imbalances' in the body are invariably blamed for illness or susceptibility to illness (see chapter 5 for a summary of the philosophies of the latter alternative healing systems).

Certainly, the popularity of CAM has accelerated in Northern Europe, the United States and Australia over the last decade, and recent surveys have indicated that over half of general practitioners in the UK offer some form of complementary therapy while one in four people in Britain have tried some form of CAM (Dobson 2003). Although the general public, and increasingly health professionals in hospitals and GP surgeries, progressively view CAM as having an important place in health maintenance and prevention, also in many chronic conditions, the role of CAM in life-threatening illnesses such as cancer is far more controversial. Alternative healing systems are still regarded with suspicion and hostility, as in the recent controversies over evidence-based research in homeopathy, but the situation in the UK and in other biomedically dominated healthcare systems regarding complementary therapies is rather different. In the UK, for instance, osteopathy and chiropractic are often integrated into the mainstream healthcare system and may even be provided free of charge. Sceptics argue that, rather than showing a real willingness to integrate, the more chronic, difficult-to-treat conditions such as persistent lower back pain are readily surrendered by biomedicine (Cant and Sharma 1999).

Integrated models of health and illness

The divide between physical and mental illness also historically reinforces hierarchical divisions within medicine, since anything that is classified as a mental illness is and always has been consistently stigmatized and marginalized (Cant and Sharma 1999). However, epidemiological patterns reveal increasing prevalence; for instance, recent estimates claim that at least 25 per cent of GP consultations in the UK are prompted by psychological symptoms and that 20 per cent or more of UK adults have a recognizable medically defined *mental* disorder (Mental Health Foundation 2005). These mainly comprise anxiety and depressive disorders, of which

80–90 per cent are managed (or not) in primary care rather than by the mental health services. Moreover, behaviours which are now perceived as being major health risks, such as smoking, overeating, alcohol and substance abuse, attempted suicide, violence, accidents and sexually transmitted diseases, inevitably have important emotional components. Since the 1980s the *biopsychosocial* model gained popularity amongst physicians as its multicausal definition allowed for the variety of perspectives to be taken into account in diagnosis and treatment, implying an inherently multidisciplinary approach. However, this model has also been criticized for not fully addressing mind/body dualism as the patient can still be compartmentalized by the physician addressing biomedical symptoms and the psychologist/psychiatrist the psychosocial element. More recently, the combined shift towards both holism and interdisciplinarity in healthcare practice has resulted in *integrated models* becoming the preferred consensual term for both practitioners and theorists (Wade and Halligan 2004). Table 1.3 charts the paradigm shift in models of health which renders the labels of physical and mental illnesses as outdated and redundant.

Table 1.3 A paradigm shift in models of health and illness

Biomedical model	Integrative model
Mechanistic	Holistic
Body–mind dualism/ reductionism	Interaction between body/mind
Single fundamental cause of illness	Multicausality
Isolated individual	Socially connected individual
Treatment	Treatment
• Curative 'magic bullet' approach	• Appropriate interventions (may be biological/ psychosocial)
• Pharmaceutical/ technological interventions	• Management
	• Preventive: health maintenance
Focus on acute illness	Focus on long-term health
	Allows for chronic illness

Thus, the critique of biomedicine, with its emphasis on high technology, cure and 'body machines' (see table 1.3) has developed alongside the decline of infectious diseases, at least in the 'West'. Across North America, Northern and Western Europe and Australasia, infectious disease as a cause of mortality and morbidity has largely been replaced by degenerative and 'lifestyle' illnesses, including cancer, diabetes, vascular disease, arthritis and the dementias. Both biomedicine and social sciences have been challenged by these illnesses, characterized as they are by multifactorial aetiologies and complex mind–body relationships, resulting in the re-evaluation of traditional categories, formulations and management strategies. The biomedical model also tends to rely uncritically on EBM, creating polarization between EBM and VBM. In turn, this polarization limits understanding of the subjective illness experience, and subsequently of effective treatments, especially in the case of chronic illness. Social sciences and humanities associated with medicine, particularly medical sociology, philosophy/bioethics and health psychology, have shaped modern ideas about health and illness and over the course of the twentieth century formed a major challenge to the narrow philosophical grounding of biomedicine. The combined impact of these factors has prompted critical developments in medical education, reflected in the UK in the rise of the 'new' medical schools and in radical changes in the medical curriculum including an unprecedented emphasis on the social sciences and ethics (General Medical Council 1993, 2002; Greenhalgh and Hurwitz 1998). In addition the raised professional and academic status of allied professions including nursing, social work and occupational therapy, together with established social science disciplines such as medical sociology and health psychology, has contributed to make health and illness studies one of the most vibrant and important theoretical and empirical arenas in modern life.

Undoubtedly the biomedical model, with its focus on isolated individuals, external pathogens and 'magic bullet' cures, has achieved so much in fighting infectious disease produced by single organisms such as tuberculosis, smallpox and cholera (and continues to do so although this has to be qualified contextually in the 'developing world'), and the development of EBM has reinforced the need for safe ethical practice without iatrogenic consequences.

Nevertheless, it is impossible to disregard the severe limitations of this model in relation to the contemporary patterning of health and illness, as in the case of:

- diseases associated with older age, such as arthritis, Alzheimer's and Parkinson's disease
- chronic illnesses which may persist across the whole life course without 'cure', but require adaptation and management, such as diabetes, chronic pain
- complex 'disorders of late modernity' such as anorexia, depression, eating and anxiety disorders and including the proliferation of 'acronym' disorders such as IBS, CFS, ADHD
- multifactorial degenerative illnesses such as cancer, chronic obstructive pulmonary disease (COPD) and vascular disease, which now account for the vast majority of contemporary mortality figures in the 'west'.

Markedly, these disorders and conditions of contemporary modern life feature emotional as well as physiological characteristics, but the dominance of biomedicine means that physicians may be confused and frustrated by bodily symptoms without signs, and by signs without demonstrable pathology. Thus, if aetiology is not organic it must be psychiatric, and it is this reductionist translation into the categories of physical and mental illness which causes such consternation to the critics of this model. As McWhinney, Epstein and Freeman (1997) assert, mind/body dualism 'runs like a fault line through medicine' with each side having its own textbooks, clinical methods and nosology. Although embodiment has been the topic of much social science interest over the past twenty years, concepts have remained generally abstract. More recently, empirical research has begun to address embodiment, but the 'emotionally expressive' body within health and illness remains relatively unexplored. Progress has been stalled by the dominance of Cartesian dualism in biomedicine, based on the separation of mind and body, and the conception of 'body machines'.

In particular, these illnesses of late modernity feature multifactorial aetiologies and complex mind–body relationships which require traditional categories, formulations and management strategies to be re-evaluated; hence the turn to more holistic models of health and illness (see table 1.3) which are now permeating medical education and practice. In order to begin to address the impact of a more integrated account of health and illness, chapter 2 begins by considering how the difficulties outlined in the artificial separation of mind and body translate into concepts of 'stress'.

2
'Stress': The Key to Mind/ Body Medicine?

Key concepts: stress, biopsychosocial models, health capital, emotional management, emotion work, dramaturgical stress, mind/body/society models, integrated medicine

Concepts of stress

> Stress – the strain that remains when tension is not success-fully overcome.' (Antonovsky 1979: 3)

Crucial to understanding the mind/body health and illness connection is the concept of stress, which can be defined in many different ways. Like health, stress is a contested concept which has a multitude of meanings and interpretations across the lay and clinical divide, but even though definition may be difficult, it does not necessarily mean that it is not a useful concept.

Paradoxically there is no medically defined *condition* of stress, yet stress is cited as a risk factor in many life-threatening diseases, as well as a possible cause of the ever-increasing clinically diagnosable conditions of late modernity. Stress management experts would contend that by giving a name to unhappiness, the causes of stress and related physical problems can help in our understanding of how to combat unhappiness, and to treat it when it does arise. Even the hardened cynics of phenomena such as 'work stress' acknowledge that stress is 'real' insofar as it has real consequences for those who face problems at work (Wainwright and Calnan 2002). In everyday conversation it is common to hear of people being 'stressed out', 'strung up', 'burnt out', and a proliferation of similar idioms reflect the profound impact of stress in contemporary life. This apparent ubiquity implies that we need to understand not only what stress is, or rather what it represents, but also the reasons why it has become such a dominant part of modern culture, and what its implications are for us as individuals and as a society.

Perhaps the most popularly accepted definition of stress describes the process of experiencing demands which exceed the resources of an individual, or in other words a perceived loss of control which inevitably has negative consequences. However, the idea that stress is always negative is questionable. Hans Selye, one of the founding fathers of stress research, maintained that 'stress is not necessarily something bad: the stress of exhilarating, creative successful work is beneficial, while that of failure, humiliation or infection is detrimental' (Selye 1956: 141). He also believed that the biochemical effects of stress would be experienced irrespective of whether the situation was positive or negative. Many joyful or celebratory events such as giving birth, achieving work promotion or academic qualifications, buying a new house may be seen as extremely stressful, but far from injurious to health or wellbeing. Indeed a certain amount of 'positive stress' may be desirable as stimulus and encouragement.

One emerging school of thought suggests that much of what is described as 'stress' is merely 'everyday' unhappiness and 'normal' disappointment (Craib 1994; Summerfield 2001), or as Bauman so succinctly puts it, 'the lost link between objective affliction and subjective experience' (2000: 211). In other words, for many modern-day commentators, the *stress discourse* indicates a 'lack of resilience' in modern life; so being *stressed* in this model is actually a normal, even desirable human experience, warranting no place for investigations of health and illness (Furedi 2004). This critique deserves due consideration, and will be discussed in more detail throughout this book, but it is nevertheless the lived reality of many people that disturbing emotions such as fear, anger and anxiety can be experienced in emotionally and physically traumatic ways, as in the following accounts from Nathan and Rachel, who both agreed to be interviewed as part of a study exploring lay concepts of pain (Bendelow 2000).

Case study: Nathan

Aged 25, Nathan was unsure of his family background and ethnicity, as most of his childhood had been spent in children's homes, with some short-term fostering. He wanted be a theatre designer and, despite leaving school at 16, had studied part-time at a local university and obtained a degree in the subject. He was currently unemployed, although picked up occasional acting parts, and tried to sell his paintings to local galleries. He lived in what he described as 'elegant squalor' in a squat in northwest London with his wife and an artist friend; the interview took place in a room full of canvases. Nathan had experienced a variety of health problems over the last year, including a hernia, frequent bouts of influenza, and a varicose vein on a testicle needing removal. We had been discussing Nathan's questionnaire response to an item asking respondents to describe their worst pain experience. He had written about toothache, which had persisted over a whole weekend, as he was unable to get emergency treatment, and felt so out of control that he ended up punching his fist into a picture and cut his hand open. As we talked, Nathan revealed that lately he had been suffering from what he described as 'panic attacks', which were becoming much worse, and had an extremely debilitating effect upon his life as he so vividly describes:

> I have been experiencing what has been described as panic attacks but I don't know if it's a really suitable description, the first time it was like a depersonalization and once that occurred, for the next four or five days, whatever I did when I picked up a cup or looked in the mirror, I felt totally separate from whatever was going

on – it was like an inner terror . . . it's gone and it's come back and I've been seeing a psychologist for seven months and I'm going to have acupuncture. It always comes at completely illogical times, it's not as if I'm a depressive – I don't have a recurrent theme in my head. It can come when I'm feeling incredibly happy and relaxed, that's what's so frustrating about it . . . because the whole time I've been convinced it's something physical, obviously, because it makes it that much easier to bear, and more respectable somehow – I mean I still think maybe I've got a chemical imbalance or I ought to try maybe more homeopathic things, I don't know that much about it but it just seems like sitting in a room with some bloke talking about my childhood doesn't bear any kind of relation to the kind of feelings I'm going through. And I mean it is like a physical pain at times, it's like a vice on my temples and an incredible pressure on my head that it does produce a headache but essentially it's just a brooding feeling within the skull. That's why, I mean I've been to see doctors and GPs and I really wanted to have a brain scan and all these things. The longer it's gone on the more I've sort of come to terms with it – I always carry diazepam, it's like a safety measure – I very rarely use it but it's nice to know it's there.

Nathan had reluctantly come to accept that what he was describing could be interpreted as physical manifestations of stress, but was very insistent that he would have preferred his distress to have a physical cause, which he would have felt to be more 'respectable', than the presumably emotional/ psychological nature of the condition.

Case study: Rachel

Aged 34 and describing herself as 'white British', Rachel had trained as a general nurse and midwife before taking a higher degree in community health, and was working full-time as an immunization facilitator when she took part in the pain study. She had been discussing what she had considered to be her most painful experience, namely an incident in hospital in the middle of wound treatment; the dressing for a skin graft on her leg was being changed and she was neglected by hospital staff leaving the wound exposed for around half an hour. She had injured her leg in a motorcycle incident in Bangladesh two years previously. As well as the trauma of travelling back to England with a smashed leg, she had undergone extensive treatment and plastic surgery, but felt that this incident was made worse by the neglect and humiliating treatment by the nursing and medical staff. During the course of the interview, she discussed how definitions of pain should be conceptualized in much wider terms, and that previously, as a health professional, she had always defined it in narrower sensory terms. However, the recent traumatic breakdown of her long-term relationship had caused her much anguish and she felt that the emotional pain she had to endure as a consequence was far worse than any physical pain she had experienced:

> I think you can see *physical* pain as a result of *emotional* trauma . . . like you asked how you see things in your life affecting your health and one thing I put was things going well within the primary relationship and – I've recently split up from my partner in the last few weeks and I know that some of the *emotional* pain I've had from that has been experienced *physically* in terms of um – really aching inside all around the stomach and – I'm sure that's an *emotional* thing but I can feel it *physically* . . . I think that – it may be different for different people but I know that *emotional* pain and stress manifest themselves in *physical* ways in me and I can recognize my stress responses and I do get sort of aching inside and I come out in cold sores. On one occasion I came out in an incredible itchy rash and as soon as you start dealing with the stress that's provoking that, then it stops. There's probably something in between that, it's a two-step thing . . . but the *emotional* pain goes on longer – I think it's somehow worse than a *physical* pain because that is usually comprehensible, logical and there's a certain amount of control – you can get your head round it but I'd rather go through half an hour of what I described happened to me in hospital than two months of what I've just been through.

Both Nathan's and Rachel's accounts illustrate the 'lived physicality' of emotional stress and distress, and reveal the inseparability of mind and body.

Stress and ill health

Although stress may be understood in many different ways, there seems to be widespread acceptance that negative emotions cause stress, resulting in bodily responses developing, often unhealthy *fight or flight* responses such as hyperventilation, digestive disturbances and muscle tension. In turn, these responses may heighten risk of illness, since stressed individuals are more likely to exhibit altered and unhealthy eating and sleeping habits and engage in heavier consumption of alcohol and other potentially harmful substances (Marshall, Davis and Sherbourne 2000). Prolonged exposure to an environment of inappropriate levels of physical and emotional exhaustion in which the body is in a constant state of fight or flight arousal drains energy reserves and may lead to breakdown.

Both clinically and in lay terms, there is often a distinction between stress symptoms and those symptoms which may indicate serious underlying physical or mental illness requiring referral to appropriate clinical professionals. In other words stress may or may not infer illness, but can be viewed as a precursor to the process of becoming ill. There is a prolific literature and industry devoted to stress management, which manifests in a variety of self-help formats, from textbook manuals to Internet websites, and is accessible through privately paid mental health or complementary therapists, or even sometimes through state-subsidized healthcare at GP surgeries or mental health units.

The manuals and websites also present a logically ordered sequence of diagnostic procedure that would ideally take place, thus:

> When the doctor suspects that a patient's illness is connected to stress, he or she will take a careful history that includes stressors in the patient's life (family or employment problems,

other illnesses, etc.). Many physicians will evaluate the patient's personality as well, in order to assess his or her coping resources and emotional response patterns. There are a number of personality inventories and psychological tests that doctors can use to help diagnose the amount of stress that the patient experiences and the coping strategies that he or she uses to deal with them. Stress-related illness can be diagnosed by primary care doctors, as well as by those who specialize in psychiatry. The doctor will need to distinguish between adjustment and anxiety or mood disorders, and between psychiatric disorders and physical illnesses (e.g. thyroid activity) that have psychological side effects. (Frey 2007)

Table 2.1 presents a general picture of the way concepts of stress are presented in the self-help literature widely available on the Internet. We can understand stress as a general concept describing a 'load' on the system, usually external, but with humans it is internal, and a *stressor* is a specific problem, issue, challenge or personal conflict which may be external or internal. Then a stress *reaction* is an individual response to a given stressor (physiological, behavioural, emotional, cognitive, signs and symptoms). In this model, strain is the

Table 2.1 Definitions of stress in self-help advice

Stress	'load' on the system, usually external, whereas with humans it is internal	physical emotional cognitive behavioural
Stressor	specific problem, issue, challenge, personal conflict which may be external or internal	physiological bioecological emotional/ psychological social
Stress reaction	individual response to stressor(s)	signs and symptoms
Strain	the prolonged impact of the stressor on the system (overload)	precursor to illness

prolonged impact of a stressor on the system (overload), fatigue, and precursor to illness.

All of the following may be involved in stress, strain and stress reactions:

- **Physical signs and symptoms of stress** including but not limited to: increased heart rate; pounding heart; elevated blood pressure; sweaty palms; tightness of the chest, neck, jaw and back muscles; headache; diarrhoea; constipation; urinary hesitancy; trembling, twitching; stuttering and other speech difficulties; nausea; vomiting; sleep disturbances; fatigue; shallow breathing; dryness of the mouth or throat; susceptibility to minor illness, cold hands, itching; being easily startled; chronic pain and dysponesis.
- **Emotional signs and symptoms of stress** including but not limited to: irritability, angry outbursts, hostility, depression, jealousy, restlessness, withdrawal, anxiety, diminished initiative, feelings of unreality or overalertness, reduction of personal involvement with others, lack of interest, tendency to cry, being critical of others, self-deprecation, nightmares, impatience, decreased perception of positive experience opportunities, narrowed focus, obsessive rumination, reduced self-esteem, insomnia, changes in eating habits and weakened positive emotional response reflexes.
- **Cognitive/perceptual signs and symptoms of stress** including but not limited to: forgetfulness, preoccupation, blocking, blurred vision, errors in judging distance, diminished or exaggerated fantasy life, reduced creativity, lack of concentration, diminished productivity, lack of attention to detail, orientation to the past, decreased psychomotor reactivity and coordination, attention deficit, disorganization of thought, negative self-esteem, diminished sense of meaning in life, lack of control/need for too much control, negative self-statements and negative evaluation of experiences.
- **Behavioral signs and symptoms of stress** including but not limited to: increased smoking, aggressive behaviours (such as while driving), increased alcohol or drug use, carelessness, undereating, overeating, withdrawal, listlessness,

hostility, accident-proneness, nervous laughter, compulsive behaviour and impatience.

Stressors may be external or internal, including but not limited to:

* Physiological, e.g. infection, hunger, injury.
* Bioecologial: e.g. climate, pollution, food additives.
* Emotional: e.g. thoughts, values, beliefs, attitudes, perceptions.
* Social: e.g. socioeconomic status, housing, caring roles, work, human rights violations.

Ultimately, failure to respond appropriately to early signs of stress, and working continually at inappropriate levels of pressure, may result in tiredness, exhaustion, burnout, illness or even death (Arroba and James 1992: 107), and stress-related illnesses are now the most common reason given for absence from work. So whether or not stress is a 'real' medical condition,

> the very fact that the category has such a powerful and persistent hold on both the public and the scientific imagination suggests that it must partially grasp the reality of lived experience. (Wainwright and Calnan 2002: 44)

As such, it is perhaps the most important link between mind and body in health and illness, needing to be fully researched and understood across the lay–professional spectrum, and to be investigated as seriously by scientific evidence-based medicine as genetic or biological causes.

Biopsychological models of stress

In scientific discourse, stress has traditionally been theorized as being located in individual biology or psyche, as in Cannon's fight-and-flight model (1929) and the elaboration of mechanistic and homeostatic models which invoke images of 'tension' and 'pressure'. This early research on stress established the existence of the now familiar fight-or-flight response, and Cannon demonstrated the process whereby if an organism experiences a shock or perceives a threat, it quickly releases hormones, in particular adrenaline, as a survival mechanism to enable it to run faster and fight harder. In humans, as in other animals, this hormonal release acts physiologically to increase heart rate and blood pressure, delivering more oxygen and blood sugar to power important muscles. Sweating increases in an effort to cool these muscles and help them stay efficient, and blood is diverted away from the skin to the core of our bodies, reducing blood loss if we are damaged (hence the characteristic pallor of alarm). Additionally this hormonal response focuses attention onto the threat, to the exclusion of everything else, which additionally improves our ability to survive life-threatening events.

In modern life, however, it is not the case that only life-threatening events trigger this reaction: it can be experienced merely by something unexpected or something that frustrates our goals. When the threat is small, our response is minimal and may even go unnoticed among the many other distractions of a stressful situation. As Marshall et al. (2000) elaborate in their model of stress, this impressive mobilization of the body for survival also has negative consequences, as it produces a state of excitability, anxiousness and irritability, which reduces the ability to work effectively and interact with others. Inevitably, it is invariably the case that bodily trembling and pounding hearts are not compatible with precise, controlled skills, intense concentration and sound decision making. Stress can be understood as a response to an inappropriate level of demands or pressure placed upon an individual beyond his or her capacity to cope effectively. Most models suggest that the resulting physiological, behavioural and psychological processes may directly influence health and there are well-established implications for illness and disease through physiological mechanisms including the autonomic nervous and neuroendocrine systems, which in turn influence immune, gastrointestinal, neuromuscular and cardiovascular function. Acute activation of these systems is known to precipitate short-term adaptive physiological changes as well as a whole range of somatic symptoms (e.g. rapid heart rate, increased perspiration, gastrointestinal motility) that may be experienced as symptomatic of ill health. Although physiological activation has short-term adaptive benefits such as motivation and drive, chronic activation of these systems is believed to enhance vulnerability to cardiovascular, metabolic, immune-related and other diseases as well as changes in the central nervous system and the structure of the brain itself (Marshall et al. 2000).

Selye's influential adaptation model (1956) describes stress as an ongoing process of adaptation which follows the sequence of:

alarm → resistance → exhaustion

In this model, temporary stress can cause a useful adaptation as long as the body can return to homeostasis. However, the experience of chronic stress may prevent homeostasis and lead to ill health, as in the following sequence:

stress → fatigue → exhaustion→ lowered immunity → ill health

Recent research by Lundberg (2006) emphasizes how perceived stressors, both objective and subjective, impact upon bodily systems, sleep and breathing patterns, cognitive functioning, healing processes and immune systems, citing research evidence that has claimed for some time that chronic stress contributes to life-threatening conditions such as coronary heart disease (Jenkins 1976) and cancer (Schmale and Iker 1971) as well as to non-specific morbidity including colds and influenza (Aneshensel and Huba 1983).

Most biologically orientated models are homeostatic in the sense that they imply that long-term health maintenance depends upon a balanced combination of anabolic processes with necessary resources to maximize the *benefits* of stress, namely energy mobilization and positive stimuli, whilst simultaneously allowing for restoration, healing and regeneration.

Mind/body/society models of stress

It seems reasonable that a certain degree of stress is a normal part of a living organism's response to the inevitable changes in its physical or social environment, and that positive, as well as negative, events can generate stress as well as negative occurrences. Along the spectrum, stress can be seen as positive, in the sense of providing drive and motivation, as well as negative – as both health-promoting and health-damaging – and the models described above convey to some extent the complex intertwining of emotion and embodiment.

However there is still often a distinction made between stress-related *physical* illnesses, such as irritable bowel syndrome, heart attacks and chronic headaches, which are thought to result from the long-term overstimulation of a part of the nervous system that regulates the heart rate, blood pressure and digestive system, and stress-related *emotional* illness which may result from complex responses to major changes in one's life situation, including events such as marriage, attaining educational or professional qualifications, becoming a parent, becoming unemployed or retired. The role of sociocultural factors gains increasing recognition in stress research as being a major factor in stress-related illness (Brown and Harris 1978, Thoits 1995) and has become popularized as life event theory, as espoused in the self-help literature (see table 2.2).

Although this research adds a very important dimension to our understanding of reactions to stress, it tends to problematize the individual response, which is frequently described as *inadequate* or *inappropriate*. Clinically, psychiatrists often

Table 2.2   **Top ten most stressful life events**

1. Death of spouse
2. Divorce
3. Marital separation
4. Jail term or death of close family member
5. Personal injury or illness
6. Marriage
7. Loss of job due to termination
8. Marital reconciliation or retirement
9. Pregnancy
10. Change in financial status

Source: Medical Encyclopaedia (www.answers.com)

use the term *adjustment disorder* to describe this type of illness, and as we will see in chapter 3, there is considerable controversy as regards the pathologization of reactions to highly distressing events and trauma.

Measuring and encompassing the influence of social factors in this process is inevitably highly complex if we accept that the causes of stress can include any event or occurrence that a person considers a threat to his or her coping strategies or resources. As we have seen, stress-related disease is thought to result from excessive and prolonged demands on an organism's coping resources and the symptoms of stress are not easily divided into mental or physical. In the workplace, stress-related illness is often termed *burnout* – a loss of interest in or ability to perform one's job due to long-term high stress levels which may involve a whole range of symptoms across the physical–emotional spectrum. Whether in the public or private sphere, the world of work is increasingly presented as a source of stress, according to the Health and Safety Executive (HSE 2008):

- The 2006/7 survey of Self-reported Work-related Illness (SWI 06/07) prevalence estimate indicated that around 530,000 individuals in Britain believed in 2006/7 that they were experiencing work-related stress at a level that was making them ill.
- The 2007 Psychosocial Working Conditions (PWC) survey indicated that around 13.6 per cent of all working individuals thought their job was very or extremely stressful.
- The annual incidence of work-related mental health problems in Britain in 2006, as estimated from the surveillance schemes, was approximately 5,900 new cases per year. However, this almost certainly underestimates the true incidence of these conditions in the British workforce. The most recent survey of self-reported work-related illness (SWI 06/07) indicates that an estimated 245,000 people first became aware of work-related stress, depression or anxiety in the previous 12 months.
- Estimates from SWI 06/07 indicate that self-reported work-related stress, depression or anxiety account for an estimated 13.8 million reported lost working days per year in Britain.

However, it may be that the demands of the workplace are excessive, which this model with its emphasis on individual pathologization is unable to encompass. Essentially, in medico-pyschological models of stress, the notion of *resources* is rarely conceptualized beyond the individual, and it is perhaps here that sociological understandings of health and illness can help to illuminate the transaction between the individual and society. The stress response results in complex biochemical changes and physical sensations, and how it is experienced is thought to be little different to how it was experienced by our ancestors.

Wainwright and Calnan (2002) have explored in some detail the concept of the *work-stress victim*, a trend that is encouraged by the media, the government, the legal system and, more recently, the medical profession. Surveys conducted by the authors among a range of different workers confirm the extent to which the discourse of work stress has been assimilated in British society. From these findings, they present the possibility that workers, by adopting the identity of work-stress victim through help-seeking from a counsellor or a doctor, may effectively relinquish sovereignty over their mental life. For some, it may be necessary that they acknowledge that they cannot cope with a stressful job. But for many, the very process of raising awareness of stress and offering 'support' may facilitate the transition from active worker to passive victim. Although the blurring of the distinction between 'coper' and 'non-coper' may reduce the stigma of failure, it may also lower expectations of resilience, and Wainwright and Calnan are sceptical of many of the assumptions of the work-stress epidemic (2002).

For example, it is generally accepted that changes in working conditions and practices over the past twenty or thirty years have had a negative effect on workers. But there can be little doubt that working lives were much more arduous, dangerous and insecure in the first half of the twentieth century, when there was no epidemic of work stress. The authors ask whether work has become harder or workers have become less resilient and concede that this straightforward question is 'surprisingly difficult to answer'. They set about trying to answer it, not only by reviewing the familiar changes in the workplace and the labour market over the past twenty years, but by placing these changes in the wider political and ideological climate that has emerged following the collapse of socialism and the transformation of the trade unions. The unions now play a central role in promoting the concept of 'work stress', together with issues of bullying and harassment in the workplace. As Wainwright and Calnan put it, 'work stress is the phenomenal form taken by antagonistic production relations in Western society at the current time' (2002: 124).

Whether or not adverse experiences at work lead 'to more serious psychological or physical health problems appears to depend upon a wide range of personal, social and cultural factors that determine an individual's resilience'. In contrast with most accounts of work-related stress, which tend to take it at face value as an epidemic disorder of the modern work place, Wainwright and Calnan (2002) emphasize the central importance of the subjective factor, of the outlook of workers themselves, in the emergence of this phenomenon. In place of the work-stress victim, they propose a 'mentally competent, emotionally resilient subject who has high expectations of human potential'.

It could be possible that stress is a *mimetic* disorder, namely a form of hysteria whereby people mimic socially acceptable ways of exhibiting distress. If so, the current interest in, and expression of, stress in the workplace may lie more in societal and subjective changes than with purely biomedical explanations. The work of Richard Wilkinson (1996) on psychosocial determinants in relation to health inequalities in particular has taken into consideration the individual's repertoire of coping resources and vulnerabilities. Wilkinson (1996) suggests that in developed countries, although health inequalities are linked to socioeconomic status, the effects of income and living standards are mediated by psychosocial pathways which are located in the social meanings attached to individual circumstances. Building on these theories, recent work by Dolan (2007) exploring health beliefs of working-class men suggests:

> the greater the perceived degree of difference in material resources . . . the more people experience various forms of

worry, stress, insecurity and vulnerability, which are translated inside the body into poorer health via the body's internal
stress systems. In addition, increased levels of stress and other
negative emotions may carry a further health penalty in terms
of increasing the likelihood of risk-taking forms of behaviour.
(Dolan 2007: 713)

Building upon the idea of health as capital, the following
model can perhaps encompass both adaptation and demand/
resource models (table 2.3) in understanding stress. In this
model, sufficiently intense perceived stress may activate physiological, behavioural and psychological processes that place
individuals at heightened risk for health problems or illness
behaviour. Long-term damage to health arises as sustained
stress leads to an inability to adapt to transient stressors;
maladaptive arousal may be low-grade but persistent.

A health capital model also allows for the fact that individuals with more resources and fewer vulnerabilities may be
less likely to perceive a given set of circumstances as stress-
provoking and that even when events are perceived as stressful, these individuals seem better able to adjust and cope. In
this way, responses to stress are not purely individual, but are
also strongly influenced by socioeconomic and behavioural
factors. Sociological theories of emotion in particular can
shed light on the relationship between social structure and

Table 2.3   A health capital model of stress

Demands = mix of life events + daily 'grind'	Resources
Biological/physical e.g. illness, risk factors demands of daily activity climate	**Biological/physical** health, geographical location physical environment
Economic/material type of work providing adequate standard of living for self/dependants	**Economic/material** survival, shelter income, education, housing
Social/cultural caring responsibilities, social roles	**Social/cultural** self-esteem, social networks

health and the phenomenological experience of illness, pain and suffering.

Emotion: the link between mind and body

Critiques of the Cartesian rationalist project have been extremely critical of the tendency in social thought to ignore the relevance of 'the body' or to viewing emotions simply as cognitive products (Bordo and Jagger 1987; Shilling 1993; Williams and Bendelow 1998) and recommend celebrating the body through an orientation which stresses the importance of desire, emotions, the affective life and corporeal intimacies (Turner 1996).

Emotion has been theorized across a variety of perspectives ranging from a deterministically biological position at one end of the spectrum to being entirely socially constructed at the other (see figure 2.1). However, it is obviously the interactionist approach, seemingly premised upon a non-dualistic ontology which seeks to unite both the biological and social realms of emotional being, which promises most.

Hochschild (1979, 1983) has played a key role in developing the *interactionist approach* to emotions (figure 2.1). Drawing on a number of interactionist theorists including John Dewey, C. Wright Mills and Erving Goffman, Hochschild developed her highly influential social theory of

BIOLOGICAL **organismic**	**interactionist**	SOCIAL **social constructionist**
biological correlates, i.e. causes of emotion 'wired in' via brain for instinct/survival	social correlates, i.e. causes of emotion found in relationships but have embodied expression	emotion not a 'thing' but is invented and expressed in differing social contexts
BIOLOGICAL *primary* SOCIAL *secondary*	SOCIAL *primary* BIOLOGICAL *secondary*	SOCIAL *primary* BIOLOGICAL *irrelevant*
emotions are universal across culture, e.g. James-Lange, Ekman	emotions are culturally relative, e.g. Goffman, Hochschild	emotions are culturally and contextually relative, e.g. early Harré, Coulter

Figure 2.1   Theories of emotion.

emotion which can be used to transcend the divides of physical 'disease' and mental 'illness'.

The interactionist approach sees emotion through the notion of the 'mindful body', as the mediatrix of phenomenological experience, social and the body politic (Scheper-Hughes and Lock 1987). Grief, for instance, is an example of emotional pain which is inseparable from its 'gut churning, nauseating experience', whilst physical pain bears within it a 'component of displeasure, and often of anxiety, sadness and anger that are fully emotional' (Leder 1984/5: 261). On the other hand, pain may also signal something positive. In this respect pain may bring us to an authentic recognition of our own limitations and possibilities. It may also be creative, not only in the sense that it is in childbirth, but also in terms of physical, emotional, artistic and spiritual achievements, or it may serve as a catalyst for much-needed changes in our lives (Leder 1984/5).

As Scheper-Hughes and Lock (1987) argue, emotions affect the way in which the body, illness and pain are experienced and are projected in images of the well and poorly functioning social and body politic: 'Insofar as emotions entail both feelings and cognitive orientations, public morality and cultural ideology, we suggest that they provide an important "missing link" capable of bridging mind and body, individual, society and body politic' (1987: 28–9). In this respect, explorations of sickness, madness, pain, disability and death are human events which are literally 'seething with emotion' (Scheper-Hughes and Lock 1987).

In her social theory of emotion, Hochschild (1983) stresses that although emotions have biological substrates, they are socially shaped and managed, therefore subject to hierarchical manipulation. She develops an *emotion management* perspective which explores the relationship between emotional experience, emotion management, feeling rules and ideology. Feeling rules are the ideological strategies we develop to deal with uncomfortable, distressing or inappropriate emotions and feelings. These may be conscious, as in Goffman's notion of unconscious *deep acting* by making oneself believe the socially desirable adaptation. Emotion management is the type of work it takes to cope with these feeling rules. Hochschild (1983) applies this mainly in the realm of gender, class and work, as for instance she argues that 'meaning-making' jobs, which tend to be more common in the middle class, put more of a premium on the individual's capacity to *do* emotion work. In this way, she maintains, each class psychologically reproduces the class structure.

The concept of *emotion work* involves the management of emotions of the individual in order to conform with the demands of the particular social situation. These include both the subjective states and more public bodily displays. Hochschild (1983) has coined the phrase 'status shields', which are the socially distributed resources that people have for protecting their sense of self in differing social situations. Again there is the theme of the division between work and home; the private sphere is seen as more appropriate than the public. The tendency towards stoicism, the traditional British 'stiff upper lip', is often portrayed with pride, and may be continually instilled throughout childhood socialization, especially for boys. However, negative consequences of the tendency to not express ourselves can occur when symptoms are ignored, either by the sufferer themselves, or those who are supposed to be caring for them. In healthcare (and no doubt in other areas of care), there is a tendency to label any sick role behaviour as 'attention seeking' at best and malingering at worst, when in fact it may be the perceptions of the carers which need examining.

An interactive theory of emotion, with its ability to bridge mind, body and society, is an exciting proposition for understanding of the role of emotion in health and illness, and the work of Peter Freund has taken the notion of dramaturgical stress forward in this area.

Dramaturgical stress: emotion in illness

As we have seen earlier in this chapter, the psychosocial causes of disease and the role of factors such as life events and difficulties, and social support in the onset of physical and mental illness, have been well established in the scientific as well as the social scientific literature, but the development of Hochschild's work by Freund has consistently held up the 'expressive body' as a common ground for the sociology of emotions, health and illness (Freund 1990, 1998; Freund, McGuire and Podhurst 2003). He maintains that the embodied self is intimately meshed with social life, thus offering endless potential for socially constructing emotions and psychological responses, and suggests that human bodies should be seen as 'acting mind-body unities' (Freund 1990: 457). Thus emotions as a form of communication can be physically expressed in motor activity (e.g. facial expression) or neurohormonally in different configurations of biological information; in other words the highly developed subjectivity of humans mediates material-physical reality (Freund 1990: 457). It is from this important set of propositions that Freund is able to develop an existential-phenomenological perspective, one which emphasizes subjectivity and the active, expressive body, in order to bridge the mind/body/society split so necessary in understanding processes of health and illness. Inevitably in this model, 'external' social structural factors such as one's position in different systems of hierarchy or various forms of social control can influence the conditions of our existence, how we respond and apprehend these conditions and our sense of embodied self. These conditions can also affect our physical functioning (Freund 1990: 461). In order to elaborate this position further, Freund draws on the writings of Hochschild on emotion work and status shields in the context of status and social control. As he notes, one's position in the social hierarchy and the activities involved in insuring social control are two features of social structure that influence feelings, which in turn influence our physiology:

> since the body is a means of expressing meaning, including socio-cultural meaning, it is not unrealistic to suppose that people might express somatically the conditions of their existence . . . cultural factors can shape the language of the body. (Freund 1990: 463)

In other words, one's position in any system of social hierarchy and the manner in which social relationships are managed both affect and are affected by biochemical states and other aspects of 'bodyliness' (Freund 1990: 465). Thus it is clear that a person's social position and status will determine the resources they have at their disposal in order to define and protect the boundaries of the self and counter the potential for 'invalidation' by powerful and significant others. Relating this more closely to key aspects of contemporary social structure, it therefore follows that those who occupy less powerful positions in the social hierarchy are at greater risk of being invalidated, of feeling instrumentally powerless, insecure, unable to speak their mind or blameworthy for the distressful feelings experienced: 'In short, an extremely powerless social status increases the likelihood of experiencing "unpleasant" emotionality or emotional modes of being' (Freund 1990: 466).

Having one's feelings ignored or termed irrational is analogous to having one's perceptions invalidated. Less powerful people, therefore, face a structurally inbuilt handicap in managing social and emotional information.

As Goffman (1959) and later Hochschild (1979, 1983) suggest, the emotion work involved in self-presentation and role playing is stressful and if, as in the widely accepted adaptation model outlined earlier, this stress becomes chronic, it may, for instance, affect neurohormonal regulation in the body. It is these forms of stress which Freund refers to as *dramaturgical stress*, and which are linked to the health capital model as social status provides *status shields* available to protect the boundaries and integrity of the self (Hochschild 1979, 1983).

Mind/body medicine and integrative models

The term mind/body medicine has been in use for some time, although still regarded with scepticism as a populist 'new-age' fad and even derided by many health professionals. It was popularized in the United States by Bernie Siegel's bestseller *Love, Medicine and Miracles* (1989) who defines the term as 'the impact of emotion on physical health'. Earlier still, the physician James Lynch reached similar but more understated conclusions in his book *The Broken Heart: The Medical Consequences of Loneliness* (1977), in which he presented evidence to demonstrate the links between cardiovascular disease and emotionally distressing life events. In particular, he uses medical technology to demonstrate emotional states, for example electro-encephalographic (ECG) patterns show dramatic improvements when a nurse holds a patient's hand. However, the lack of a biomedically acceptable evidence base, as in the case of CAM as discussed in chapter 1, means that at best this type of evidence is seen as anecdotal, at worst as irrelevant. Although it may be axiomatic to both lay and professional observers that distress causes physical problems and physical factors cause emotion, it is not necessarily easy or possible to offer scientific proof through the paradigmatic 'gold standard' of medical research, the randomized controlled trial. In specialized medical domains such as oncology, research by the Cancer UK Psychosocial Centre has been able to demonstrate the benefits of psychosocial interventions, and to show that both professional and personal support can make a difference to both the experience and the outcome of cancer trajectories (see for instance Macleod, Ross, Fallowfield and Watt 2004). Nevertheless, within conventional medicine, body–mind approaches have largely been confined to the field of psychosomatics, which is subsumed under the psychiatric rubric, classifying symptoms as 'imaginary' or not 'real', thus reinforcing rather than challenging the mental–physical and body–mind problematic.

The limits of mental/physical labels

As we saw in chapter 1, social sciences and humanities associated with medicine, particularly health psychology, medical sociology and philosophy/bioethics, have shaped modern ideas about health and illness and over the course of the twentieth century posed a major challenge to the narrow philosophical grounding of biomedicine. Rather than a crude polarization between biomedical and social models, which may exacerbate rather than alleviate the problem, the trend towards developing integrated models appears to provide a more enlightened path. The biopsychosocial model, originally attributed to Engel (1950), gained considerable currency from the 1980s onwards and, although it is criticized for overdetermining the biomedical component of aetiology and treatment, it has provided an important template to develop new holistic and integrated models.

In contemporary healthcare, even the most conventional biomedical physicians accept or would find it difficult to refute that 'real' physical events mediate mind–body connections, in the sense that emotional stimuli (through thoughts and feelings) produce physiological changes in the body. Likewise, when a coping strategy improves a physical condition, the change mechanism between talk (or method) and the illness takes place physically somewhere in the body: for instance nerves associated with thoughts change in the brain, messages are sent in the nervous system, conditions of the muscles change, hormones flow, the immune system is activated or inhibited. The health capital model of stress outlined in this chapter (table 2.3) encapsulates the multicausal multilevel interplay of biological, emotional and social factors involved in individual responses which may or may not manifest in pathology or illness without underplaying or overdetermining the role of material and psychosocial resources.

The most imaginative concepts of stress describe the problems of coping with a perceived, real or imagined threat to one's physical, mental, spiritual or emotional wellbeing, resulting in a series of physiological responses and adaptations. The limitations and inadequacies of scientific medicine in separating mind and body, reducing individuals to 'body machines', as discussed earlier, have long been a source of controversy highlighted by social scientists working within health and illness, particularly through the second-wave feminists' accounts of women's experiences of medicalization, and more recently through the burgeoning body of work on illness narratives. These critiques have influenced the turn to more holistic integrative models of health and illness, which are now permeating medical education and practice (Wade and Halligan 2004) and serve to highlight further the outmoded relevance of mental/physical labels.

3
Medically Unexplained Symptoms and 'Contested Conditions'

Key concepts: mind/body divide; MUS; somatization; psychiatriform disorders; contested conditions; social construction of illness; suffering, trauma and PTSD; childhood disorder and ADHD; 'disease mongering'; emotional health

Medicine and the mind/body divide

In the last chapter it was argued that to further understand the role of emotion and embodiment in health and illness, we need more elaborate reconceptualizations of 'stress' – as link between mind and body, and also between mind, body and society. This chapter addresses how the translation of symptoms into medically classified illnesses can be severely limited by the polarization into either mental or physical categories. Moving beyond biomedicine, a symptom can be defined as so much more than just a chemical dysfunctioning, in that it also denotes clues and indications of the embodied expression of human experience (Phillips 2006). If we accept that most systems of healing and medicine use symptoms to diagnose illness, disruption or imbalance, this leads to further problematization of the dualistic divides in understanding illness. A more integrated approach may be to take the 'lived body' or the phenomenological experience of the body as a starting point for interpreting symptoms.

As outlined in chapter 1, the reductionist features of Cartesian dualism in contemporary 'western' medicine are not only culturally and historically specific, they are also a comparatively recent phenomenon. In western medicine, holistic concepts of bodily ills have been in existence since the Ancient Greeks as emotions such as grief, pity and love were thought to reside in internal organs such the heart, liver and spleen (Phillips 2006). Until the popularity of Galenic medicine began to decline in the seventeenth century, emotion and embodiment, physical and mental symptoms were inextricably linked in aetiological concepts in western medicine, as they still are in other healing systems (see chapter 5), and hysteria was one of the most established diagnostic concepts which was able to encompass the mind/body divide.

Hysteria

Indeed, the historical emergence of the concept of hysteria is attributed to the description by Hippocrates of the infamous 'wandering womb', which when diseased or damaged was considered to move around the body uncontrollably, causing pain and distress (Martin 1987). Although Galen, the ancient Greek physician whose theories dominated western medicine until the emergence of biomedicine in the 1800s, later confirmed the uterus to be a stationary organ, the connection of hysteria with female sexual dysfunction persisted into Victorian ideology, and many would argue still persists today. Even though hysterical symptoms were understood to occur in male pathology, these were more readily seen as hypochondriacal, or to be attributed to the spleen (Phillips 2006). Furthermore, as Showalter emphasizes (1998), the equating of female sexual dysfunction and emotion with hysteria became even more pronounced throughout the eighteenth and nineteenth centuries. Foucault's deconstruction of the how the clinical gaze defined the systematic medical observation of the body drew heavily on the research on hysteria in late nineteenth-century Paris when it was defined by Charcot at Salpêtrière as a medical disorder with specified symptoms.

Social construction of illness was hinted at as the incidence of hysteria rose from 1 per cent to 17.3 per cent during Charcot's tenure, despite his insistence thus:

> It would be truly marvellous if I were thus able to create illnesses as the pleasure of my whim and caprice. But for the truth, I am absolutely only the photographer, I register what I see. (quoted in Showalter 1987: 151)

Subsequently, Freud's groundbreaking and infamous work with hysterical females addressed the bodily performativity of emotional distress, suggesting that the development of their physical symptoms such headaches, coughs and loss of voice (globus hystericus) could be interpreted as a reaction to powerlessness. Despite the entrenched sexism of the period, and other criticisms of Freud's work (including a lack of scientific credibility), the concept of hysteria has current validity as Showalter so aptly demonstrates. In the last chapter, it was suggested that the physical acting-out by the body of emotional distress, which in turn is too often caused by powerlessness, oppression and exploitation, is interpreted as stress. In other words stress can be understood as a modern-day manifestation of hysteria, which is perhaps a more socially acceptable term, without the gendered connotations. The following case study is presented as a contemporary example.

Case study: Tanya

Tanya was adopted as a baby and never knew her biological parents, only that her father was thought to be Iranian. Her adoptive father was British Caribbean, her mother white British, and she grew up in a predominantly white working-class West Midlands neighbourhood. She knew from a very early age that she was adopted and had an intense passionate relationship with her father who continually told her how much he adored her, and that he had chosen her out of all the children in the world to be his daughter, whereas her mother did not try to hide that she had never wanted to have children.

Tanya was extremely clever at school, and a high achiever all the way to postgraduate level at university, eventually becoming a high-ranking civil servant. Despite her adoptive father's bouts of heavy drinking and aggression, she remained devoted to him and was devastated when he died of cancer when she was in her early thirties. Throughout her twenties and thirties she had three long-term heterosexual relationships, but was adamant that she had no desire to marry or have children. When a five-year relationship with a younger man broke up in her early forties, his wishes to have children seemed to be a significant, if not the only, factor. After her partner left her, Tanya had severe sleep problems, experiencing some strange hallucinatory experiences, and believed her father was trying to communicate with her. She also had bouts of eating disorders, self-harming, binge-drinking, and sought out casual sexual encounters which always ended with her feeling totally abandoned.

Although she had a warm and supportive circle of friends, Tanya also became very distressed at this time about her relationship with her only relative, namely her mother, who had always been emotionally cold and withheld. Tanya had always vehemently denied that being adopted was ever a problem, and had been very cynical about therapy, but eventually sought out a therapist she felt she could trust, and who began to explore her parental relationships. Although Tanya was extremely resistant to discussing the adoption, feeling it would be disloyal to the memory of her adoptive father, after several months, her therapist was able to initiate exploration.

Whilst driving home after this first intense session, Tanya experienced strange physical sensations, literally a 'shutting down' of her bodily functions, and had to pull over and stop the car. She thinks she lost consciousness for several minutes, but managed to pull herself together enough to drive home, and immediately slept for over 12 hours.

Despite the distress experienced as a result of addressing her past, Tanya has found the therapy to be useful in gaining insights into emotions that she previously felt powerless to manage or understand, and has persevered for over a year. She no longer desires to act in a manner she now sees as being self-destructive and self-harming, and her career and her social life continue to strengthen and remain very successful. She has not since experienced anything of the same intensity after subsequent sessions, but occasionally has again experienced 'out of body' sensations (again a sense of 'closing down') after some of the encounters, or if she finds herself in social situations where she again feels alone and abandoned. However, she claims that she no longer feels frightened or alarmed by these experiences, but can contextualize them as her body 'acting out' her distress.

Somatization

Although biomedicine is typically characterized as not recognizing the relationship between body and mind, this may be overstated as there is (and always has been) some medicalized acceptance that somatic symptoms can be manifested in response to emotional or psychosocial distress, and may be a reaction to life events or social situations stressful to the individual.

Likewise it is also the case that problems with physical health may create emotional distress. There is now abundant evidence that medical and surgical patients have a high prevalence of psychiatric disorder which can be effectively treated with psychological or pharmacological methods and the development of the subspecialty of liaison psychiatry is an example of how medicine has attempted to address the interface between physical and psychological health, providing psychiatric treatment to patients attending general hospitals, whether they attend outpatient clinics or accident and emergency departments or are admitted to the ward as inpatients. In addition, it has been estimated that 20 per cent or more of UK adults have a recognizable mental disorder and that, while 80–90 per cent of mental disorder is managed (or not) in primary care, communication between primary and secondary care is patchy, and most secondary psychiatric resources are dedicated to severe and enduring mental illness (Bower and Gilbody 2005). Specific liaison psychiatry services were virtually unknown in Britain until the 1970s, but developed from a special interest group within the Royal College of Psychiatry, with a small number of specialized consultant posts, to the status of a faculty in 1997.

From the mid twentieth century, the medical specialism of psychosomatics developed in line with biomedical nosology as a branch of medicine which identified psychological factors as aetiological in causing illness and has traditionally focused on researching conditions such as irritable bowel syndrome (IBS), ulcerative colitis or hypertension, but inevitably ends up 'straddling an uneasy path between psychiatry and organic medicine' (Greco 2001: 475), with the inevitable stigmatizing of associations between psychological and bodily distress. Greco advocates as an alternative the concept of *alexithymia* (literally meaning 'without word for emotions') which, she maintains, can be understood as:

> the difficulty in distinguishing between feelings and the bodily sensations of arousal; externally orientated cognitive style, tendency to resort to action and constricted imaginative processes, evidenced by a paucity of fantasies. (Greco 2001: 473)

Seen as a series of psychobehavioural characteristics, Greco maintains that this can be a potential paradigm to advance our understanding of psychosomatic medicine because it is not a medical or psychiatric diagnosis, and does not refer to disease entity but can be considered rather as a risk factor – a link between 'quality of relations to one's self and probability of disease'. In this way, she argues, existential styles and choices can be predisposing factors in pathogenesis.

Medical classifications of somatic symptoms

The shift towards biopsychosocial models has resulted in psychosomatics becoming superseded by *somatization*, defined as 'the tendency to experience and communicate somatic distress and symptoms unaccounted for by pathological

Table 3.1 Classification of somatoform disorders

ICD-10[1]	DSM-IV[2]
Somatoform disorder requires multiple recurrent and frequently changing symptoms of 2 years duration	Somatoform disorder requires multiple recurrent symptoms over several years for which medical investigation has taken place
Undifferentiated somatoform disorder – less than 2 years of symptoms	Undifferentiated somatoform disorder
Hypochondriacal disorder persistent preoccupation with possibility of having one or more serious and progressive physical disorders	Conversion disorder
Somatoform autonomic dysfunction	Body dysmorphic disorder symptoms suggest neurological disorder e.g. blindness, deafness, numbness in limbs
Persistent somatoform pain disorder	Pain disorder
Unspecified somatoform disorder	

[1] Source: World Health Organization (1992). ICD = International Classification of Diseases and Related Health Problems
[2] Source: American Psychiatric Association (1994). DSM = Diagnostic and Statistical Manual of Mental Disorders

findings, to attribute them to physical illness, and to seek medical help for them' (Lipowski 1988). Medically, somatization is categorized as mental illness, using a range of classifications through both ICD-10 and DSM-IV systems (see table 3.1).

Despite the detail contained in the criteria, the subjectivity of diagnosis and interpretation means that prevalence in general populations may vary widely according to ICD or DSM criteria. For instance in a study of GP attenders in the UK, Fink et al. (1999) found that only 7.1 per cent of patients were diagnosed with undifferentiated somatoform disorder according to ICD-10 criteria compared to 27.3 per cent using

DSM-IV. Conversely, the ICD diagnoses of somatization disorder revealed a prevalence of 6.1 per cent compared to 1 per cent using DSM-IV.

Moreover, the classification of somatization as psychiatric disorder using these symptom lists further reinforces the mind/body divide and underplays the physicality of the symptoms. As McWhinney, Epstein and Freeman (1997) point out, what is needed is recognition that illnesses have emotional components and emotion can be a causal agent; in other words the patient should be diagnosed, not the disease. These may include the bodily components of depression, schizophrenia and other *mental* disorders as well as somatic expressions of emotional distress in conditions such as chronic pain and chronic fatigue syndrome (otherwise known as ME). More controversial are what are often termed *contested conditions*, including:

- post-traumatic stress disorder (PTSD), anxiety disorders, e.g. seasonal affective disorder (SAD) and generalized anxiety disorder (GAD)
- behavioural disorders, e.g. ADHD, eating disorders.

These and many other classified illnesses of 'late modernity' feature a broad range of reactions to stress, loss and grief, in which the clinical status of *dysthmia*, namely the display of emotion inappropriate to circumstances, is an important but value-laden component

Medically unexplained symptoms

Medically unexplained symptoms or MUS, an acronym in popular usage in the medical and social science literature, is perhaps a more neutral and less stigmatizing label than 'psychosomatic symptoms', but still identifies illnesses or syndromes which cannot be defined in terms of organic pathology and are thus seen as abnormal and low in 'illness hierarchy' (Nettleton, O'Malley, Watt and Duffey 2004). The term 'contested conditions' is used to signify illnesses of controversial scientific status (e.g. ME – myalgic encephalomyelitis, CFS – chronic fatigue syndrome, RSI – repetitive strain injury, chronic low back pain) in which the patient experiences distressing physical symptoms such as impaired mobility or coordination, intermittent paralysis, fitting, pain, fatigue, or visual disturbance, but there is usually an absence of physical signs, clinical explanation or medical diagnosis, and estimates of GP consultations in the UK prompted by emotional or psychological issues vary between 25 and 50 per cent.

Traditionally biomedicine has been unable to deal effectively with people who present in this way, creating a 'diagnostic limbo . . . which widens the gap between clinical reductions and lost metaphysics' (Williams 1984) but may be more accessible by integrative, holistic approaches. As we have seen, physical complaints do often point to physical disorders, but pain and fatigue can also be clues to psychological disturbance which manifest in distressing symptoms which also require help or intervention.

Whereas the benefits of scientific medicine, particularly in the fight against infectious disease, are invaluable, the crude reductionism of Cartesian dualism has had detrimental implications across both sides of the divide. On the one hand it has resulted in sometimes fatal misdiagnoses in the case of life-threatening conditions which may have been treatable if discerned earlier, but were dismissed as psychological symptoms of anxiety and depression. These include endocrinopathies, cancers (especially gynaecological, and those of the pancreas, lung and central nervous system), and neurological conditions such as epilepsy, multiple sclerosis and dementia. There is a well-documented body of research that reveals how stereotyped attitudes of health professionals towards gender, social class, age and ethnicity may contribute to this process of misdiagnosis and lack of investigative procedures (see for instance Helman 2001; Bendelow et al. 2002; Wilkinson 2004), and which reinforces the need for values-based medicine to be taken account of alongside evidence-based medicine.

Integrated models of healthcare have particular value in understanding and managing the complex phenomena of medically unexplained symptoms, as detailed by the flow diagram produced by Wade and Halligan (2004: 1398) (figure 3.1).

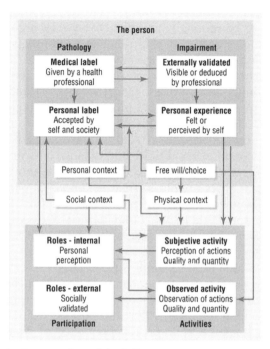

Figure 3.1 Proposed model of illness.

The acute/chronic distinction within the biomedical model can also potentially place limitations on understanding the illness experience. A primary role of medicine is often perceived as treating or alleviating pain, but what actually constitutes pain is subjective, value-laden and difficult to define objectively and empirically, relying as it does on expressivity of both bodily signs and language which are culturally embedded, subject to multiple interpretation. Medical theories of pain have traditionally concentrated upon its neurophysiological aspects, both in diagnosis and treatment, and scientific medicine reduces the experience of pain to an elaborate broadcasting system of signals, rather than seeing it as moulded and shaped by both the individual and their particular sociocultural context (an inevitable outcome of the again infamous Cartesian split between body and mind). Thus, medical understanding of pain tends to be based upon sensation or *nociception*, with the subsequent inference that it is able to be rationally and objectively measured, and this does not necessarily take emotional and cultural aspects into account. Yet as well as being a medical 'problem', the experience of pain is so much wider, lying at 'the intersection of bodies, minds and cultures' (Morris 1991: 1) and not just confined to our anatomy and physiology. The limitations of the model become especially highlighted when the acute/chronic differentiation is evoked, as chronic pain is one of the most common conditions but is most difficult to treat. It is universally acknowledged that one of the most complex and difficult types of pain to treat is *idiopathic* pain, that is, pain for which there is no established physical pathology (Melzack and Wall 1988), often termed *chronic pain syndrome*. The scientific neglect and rejection of emotional causes and risk factors in the aetiology of illness has severe implications, as in the example of chronic pain. Lay perspectives have illuminated the understandings of those working in the area of pain, most notably in the pioneering work of Melzack and Wall (1965, 1988) and Bonica (1953). Developments such as the widespread acceptance of Melzack and Wall's gate control theory of pain and the influence of the hospice movement have shifted the pain paradigm, increasing the emphasis upon cultural and psychological components and the need for a multidisciplinary approach. Social science, in particular the sociological literature on chronic illness, offers a framework for understanding the experience of chronic pain by focusing on the *person* rather than the pain.

These sociomedical models have developed a methodological focus away from epidemiological statistics towards inductive approaches using qualitative interactionist accounts of the impact of chronic illness on everyday life (Strauss 1975). Kelly and Field (1996) have emphasized the physicality of the body in chronic illness, and concepts such as biographical disruption, narrative reconstruction and illness adjustment (Williams 1984; Bury 1991; Greenhalgh and Hurwitz 1998) have been particularly valuable. In relation to the adjustment to chronic pain, Kotarba (1983) charted the process of becoming a 'pain-afflicted' person, in order to trace the continuity of personal identity. Using pain biographies he identified three stages in this process. First, there is the 'onset' stage, which is perceived to be transitory, and able to be dealt with by diagnosis and treatment. At this stage, pain is diagnosed as 'real' by physicians, preferably by being explained in physiological terms. The second stage concerns what Kotarba terms the 'emergence of doubt'. At this stage, treatment may not work, there is an increase in specialist consultations but patients still feel in control in seeking the best care available. Finally, the third stage concerns what Kotarba terms the 'chronic pain experience'. Following the shortcomings of treatment, the patient, at this stage, may return to the lay frame of reference, and seek help within the 'chronic pain subculture' (Kotarba 1983: 27). Illness narratives and phenomenological accounts have become intrinsic components of pain treatment in many pain clinics and centres, but it is essential to note that the acknowledgement of pain as 'real' by a physician is still the most important aspect in chronic pain (Glenton 2003).

Illness experience, as discussed in chapter 1, encapsulates the use of lay perspectives and narrative accounts and Hydén (1997) makes a distinction between illness as narrative, narrative about illness and narrative as illness in these accounts. As well as the use of the various types of illness narratives in data collection and research, experiences are used prolifically in literature, in popular media and increasingly as sources of lay information on the Internet.

As an example, the DipEx project, based at the University of Oxford, is a charity which has produced an award-winning website (www.dipex.org.uk) which presents lay experiences and narrative accounts from interviews with people diagnosed with a wide range of medical conditions including cancers, heart disease, diabetes, HIV, dementia and depression. Examples from DipEx interviews in the section on depression vividly describe the experiences of bodily changes and physical illness, such as upset gut or gripping head sensations, extreme tiredness or chronic fatigue.

> [When I'm in] . . . deep depression, I feel physiologically different, I have this sort of pressure around my brain, you know I feel that someone's got their hands inside there. I feel confused, I don't function properly. (DP23)

Some of the interviews describe how people had trouble getting to sleep, or staying asleep, and their chronic lack of sleep meant they were exhausted and 'shattered' during the day; others reported changes in their voice quality or in posture:

> I think people could tell from just the way I was looking, the way I, not looking after myself, the fact that I spoke in a low monotone. The, my posture, I tended to stoop and just looked generally dishevelled and not at all, not really able to cope, actually, quite despairing. (DP09)

Others reported eating disorders connected to being diagnosed with depression and these narrative accounts again reinforce the body–mind connections of illness experience.

Contested conditions and the social construction of illness

Medically unexplainable symptoms, whether of fatigue or chronic pain, may be experienced as equally severe and disabling regardless of whether the cause is physical or psychological, but its status as an 'illness' may vary considerably depending on its constitutional aetiology, and suffering is exacerbated by failure to achieve medical recognition.

Equally, in busy GP surgeries, patients with MUS who tend to consult repeatedly and have what are perceived to be 'intractable social problems' are often described as the bane of health professionals' lives, thus:

> I have about twelve hundred patients. There are some patients that I see a lot, and some I hardly see at all, and there are some I can help, and some I can't, and the patients that distress me the most are the ones I see a lot whom I can't help. We call them *heartsink* patients, for obvious reasons, and someone once reckoned that most partners in a practice have about fifty heartsinks on their books. They come in, and sit down, and they look at me, and both of us know it's hopeless, and I feel guilty and sad and fraudulent, and, if the truth be told, a little persecuted. These people don't see anyone else who can't help them, who fail them on such a regular

basis. The TV repairman who can't fix your picture, the plumber who can't stop a leak, the electrician who can't get your lights back on ... Your relationship with these people ceases, after a while, because they cannot do anything for you. But my relationship with my heartsinks will never cease. They will sit and stare accusingly at me for ever. (Hornby 2001: 128)

Conditions which are perceived to only have emotional or psychological causes and yield no physiological pathology are stigmatized further, despite a paradoxically increasing acceptance and openness as regards mental and emotional health.

According to the charity MIND, in the UK in 2006, 45 million working days were lost to stress and anxiety, which have now superseded back pain as the main cause of inability to work, resulting in £100 billion in lost output. Although, as we saw in the last chapter, *stress* has everyday parlance and validity as a concept, its status as a medical condition is contested and disputed. Alongside this phenomenon, there is public and professional concern regarding the expansion of the categories of sociopsychological disorders associated with contemporary life (Lyon 1996: 72) and increasing scepticism over the validity of these disorders as genuine 'illnesses', especially by employers and policy makers. Debate rages over cause and reality of contested conditions which are viewed as a cultural construct diagnosed on the basis of the clinical opinion and faithful belief of the practitioner. Since they cannot be clearly medically defined, they end up being manipulated by social trends and beliefs.

Mullen and Menkes (2008) suggest this phenomenon might be explained by the concept of the emergence of *psychiatriform* disorder as the obverse of somatiform disorder. As they explain, the origins of current concepts of somatization lie with ideas regarding hysterical conversion, which were long considered to mimic popular ideas about what constitutes disease, and the *conversion* symptoms of hysteria were seen to literally convert mental into physical distress, hence the origin of the clinical tendency to attribute otherwise unexplained physical symptoms to detectable mental symptomatology. However, Mullen and Menkes suggest that conversion might be better considered as conversion from unacceptable, to more acceptable, forms of distress. As such, conversion has been considered an enactment of the experience of someone with a physical disorder, a role that is helpful in managing interpersonal or intrapsychic conflict (Ziegler and Imboden 1962). Hypochondriasis, excessive worry about possible physical illness, can also be formulated with a psychiatriform variant, worry about mental ill health. As with somatoform disorders, persons who have experience of another psychiatric disorder may be most prone to develop psychiatriform symptoms. As somatoform disorders do not account for all medically unexplained symptoms, so psychiatriform presentations will not be the sole explanation for otherwise unexplained mental symptoms.

The importance of being blameless has been invoked as a reason why sufferers of fatigue syndromes insist on a non-psychiatric cause for their disability, equating 'psychiatric' with 'imaginary' or 'not real' in some way (Wessely, Hotopf and Sharpe, 1998). This may apply in a modified form in psychiatriform disorders where the patient asserts they have a psychiatric disorder but the cause lies elsewhere, for example in deep trauma (Summerfield 2001).

The medicalization of trauma, misery and madness

In chapter 1 we saw how the biomedical model prioritizes the principles of evidence-based medicine, using empirical scientific observation and recording of signs and symptoms to produce reliable diagnoses and treatment. Biomedical claims of efficacy, certainly in developed societies throughout the twentieth century, are undeniably justified in many instances, from prolonging life expectancy to improving the quality of life in the experience of physical illness and most notably in the battle for the elimination of infectious disease. Notwithstanding these gains, this model has severe limitations when dealing with symptoms without obvious physiological pathology, and is particularly challenged in the translation of emotional distress and disorder into mental illness.

The emergence of psychiatry as a medical specialism was instigated by Kraeplin to systematically organize symptoms of emotional disorder into similar independent observable categories. The development of clinical diagnostics in psychiatry, and in particular the *Diagnostic Statistical Manual*, attempted to ensure the 'neutrality' of the scientist/medic through empirical observation and by resisting the impulse to influence the truth or 'naturalness' of symptoms. However, the vexed question of the value-laden nature of interpreting symptoms which are unable to be scientifically 'measured' (unlike high cholesterol or low insulin levels) continues to haunt the conceptualization of illness with emotional content and subsequent provision of healthcare. Subsequently, psychiatry has continually been under the scrutiny of *social constructionist* critiques, which question the subjectivity involved in making a diagnosis, from within the specialism, as well as from without (see Pilgrim 2005: 149–53). This construction of mental disorder can be identified in three differing and distinct ways:

1. *Conceptual analysis* looks at coherence of concepts, for example the causes of a disorder (Szasz 1962). A classic example of the social construction of illness that is often cited is homosexuality, which was a DSM classification until 1973.
2. *Frame analysis* inspects how behaviours are socially negotiated by parties in interaction, as in Goffman's critique in *Asylums* (1963).
3. *Deconstruction*: this approach raises apprehensions about social negotiation of reality and questions whose interests are being served. Anti-psychiatrists such as R.D. Laing (1959) questioned the validity of the diagnosis of schizophrenia, suggesting that symptoms were produced by a process of family scapegoating.

Throughout history, the mentally disorderd have always been socially and legally marginalized as citizens. Since the eighteenth century, under English common law, land could be confiscated from those deemed either lunatics (*non compos mentis*) or idiots (*purus idiota*) by a jury of twelve (Scull 1993). In the first half of the twentieth century there was an administrative and geographical separation of those termed mentally ill and mentally defective. The term 'mentally defective/deficient' included congenital imbecility and feeble-mindedness and these were cared for in chronic institutions whose main function was training. In contemporary UK society, under the more generic but still contested term of disability, care and treatment is completely separate from that of those designated as mentally ill who are cared for in mental hospitals, the reformed Victorian asylum. Reaching their peak between the 1950s and the 1970s, the criteria for hospital beds for the mentally ill included 'morally deficient', but the aim was cure through medical treatment, often administered involuntarily with the aid of the 1953 and 1983 Mental Health Acts. Distinctions have always been made between psychotic and neurotic manifestations of mental disorder, with the former signifying a rupture with reality, however reality may be defined, which of course is much debated. Psychotic illness, with its association with dangerousness, defined by the Mental Health Act (1983) as the propensity to harm self or others, tends to be categorized as serious mental illness (SMI) and, despite the closure of many of the old asylums and mental hospitals throughout the 1980s and 1990s, is largely treated through psychiatric units and mental health teams. Busfield (2001) provided a helpful distinction between disorders of thought, emotion and behaviour and contemporary mental healthcare practice which can be translated into patterns of diagnosis and healthcare in contemporary Britain (see table 3.2).

As table 3.2 indicates, neurotic disorders are largely subsumed under the disorders of emotion rubric and, on the one hand, there is more apparent openness about conditions such as reactive (not psychotic) depression, anxiety disorders and even of the range of addictive behaviours. On the other hand, despite the increased openness, knowledge and information, conditions which are contested as illnesses compete alongside other constrained resources, and inevitably the mental health services and, to an even greater degree, the substance misuse services remain low priority, much as they always have been.

Table 3.2 Diagnosis and treatment of emotional disorders in contemporary Britain

Disorder category[1]	Diagnosis	Treatment provider	Nature of treatment
Thought	Serious mental illness, e.g. schizophrenia, bipolar disorder, psychotic depression	Referral mainly through GP or primary care to Mental Health Services (hospital and community care) or private clinics	Psychotropic drugs and depot injections Physical treatments, e.g. ECT, brain surgery Behavioural and psychodynamic therapies
Emotion	Anxiety and depressive disorders ADHD, eating and sleep disorders	80–90% primary care (GPs) Some specialist referral on NHS or private consultations	Pharmaceuticals: mainly SSRIs, Ritalin etc. Behavioural and psychodynamic therapies
Behaviour	Substance misuse and addictions, e.g. drugs, alcohol Sex offenders	Outside mainstream NHS healthcare, specialist services, some self-referral and private clinics	Detoxification regimes Behavioural and psychodynamic therapies

[1] Source: after Busfield (2001)

Trauma and post-traumatic stress disorder

Interest in how far physical or psychiatric disorder may be a result of living in a particular form of economic and political organization or domestic environment can be traced back to Marx's and Engels' concern with the social relations of capitalism, and with the links between these and individual health and wellbeing. Whilst recognizing the potential in terms of progress and civilization of the (then embryonic) new economic system, Marx predicted the detriment of health and wellbeing which alienation, the result of inevitable class exploitation, would produce:

> Within the capitalist system all methods for raising the social productiveness of labour are brought about at the cost of the individual labourer; all means for the development transform themselves into means of domination over, and exploitation of, the producers; they mutilate the labourer into a fragment of a man, degrade him to the level of an appendage to a machine, destroy every remnant of charm in his work, and turn it into hated toil; they estrange him from the intellectual potentialities of the labour process in the same proportion as science is incorporated in it as an independent power; they distort the conditions under which he works, subject him during the labour process to a despotism the more hateful for its meanness, they drag his wife and child beneath the wheels of the juggernaut of capital. (Marx 1906–1909 1: 708)

Despite fundamental differences in the two conceptions of society, similar concerns can be found in the works of Durkheim, most famously in *Suicide* (1897), where the concept of anomie was used to identify the social causes of suicide by relating their rates in different social groups to social characteristics of those groups.

Wilkinson (2004) advocates the necessity to take on board how emotional qualities of empathy, compassion and pity must constitute part of our understanding of risk perception and to subsequently frame social responses to 'risk' more as reaction to human pain and suffering.

While suffering has always been part of the experience of humanity, we cannot impassively accept this as a normal and inevitable part of our human condition. This is because suffering hurts too much. The problem with suffering is that it involves us in far *too much* pain. The pain of suffering so dominates our senses that it cannot be simply ignored or blithely returned to its proper place. It is all at once excruciating and overwhelming, and as such it is entirely unacceptable. It must be fought against (Wilkinson 2004: 2).

Medicalized responses to pain are ambivalent about the role of suffering in measuring and evaluating pain (Bendelow

2006), and there is a tendency for suffering to be subsumed under the psychiatric rubric as *trauma*, a term traditionally ascribed to the after-effects of experiencing very extreme events such as natural disaster and war. Experiences of trauma began to be medicalized during the twentieth century, influenced by Freudian concepts of hysteria. Traditional psychiatric diagnoses and treatment were challenged by middle-class British officers displaying symptoms of shellshock after their horrendous experiences in the First World War, but post-traumatic stress disorder (PTSD) is thought to have become a credible psychiatric diagnosis after the Vietnam war (Summerfield 2001). Summerfield points out that the disorder is constructed from sociopolitical concepts rather than psychiatric observations, and his critique of the development of PTSD as an illness challenges the twin assumptions that a psychiatric diagnosis constitutes a disease and that distress or suffering automatically implies a psychopathology.

> Post-traumatic stress disorder is the diagnosis for an age of disenchantment. Today there is often more social utility attached to expressions of victimhood than to 'survivorhood'; this is perhaps the reverse of 50 years ago. (Summerfield 2001: 322)

He claims that since the condition was given medical legitimation, trauma is conflated with any form of distress, rather than a reaction to extreme events, and rewards 'medicalized victims rather than feisty survivors'.

The clinical criteria involve mood anxiety and sleep patterns, common to many other psychiatric disorders, but given the hierarchies of stigma across the range of contested conditions, PTSD has higher prestige than many and is subsequently a more desirable diagnosis.

For example, the meaning of trauma in the conventional western context was resisted in Liebling's extraordinary study of Bagandan women who had experienced civil war in Uganda through sexual violations, multiple rapes, impregnation and destruction of foetuses. These extreme acts of sexual transgression are believed to have caused a crisis of identity in Bagandan women and men, but in this context war trauma was understood as a breakdown in cultural identity, manifested in psychological, social, cultural and physical effects, which are integrated and inseparable, not split between mind/body and society (Liebling-Kalifani 2004; Liebling-Kalifani, Marshall, Ojiambo-Ochieng and Nassozi 2007; Liebling-Kalifani, Ojiambo-Ochieng, Marshall, et al. 2008). However, this study reveals how women war survivors reconstructed their identities by taking on male roles as well as engaging in collective activities. Their ability to voice their experiences as a political act of resistance resulted in a shared identity and a decrease in reported levels of depression. For instance, at the end of a heartrending interview in which a woman described experiences of horrendous sexual savagery, she was asked what could happen to make her life improve. Her poignant but starkly simple reply to request 'a goat' does not belittle the severity of her dreadful experience, but perhaps supports Summerfield's thesis that she is not 'ill' as a result of her experience, she is indeed 'a feisty survivor'. In contrast, Liebling-Kalifani found that the men in the study largely turned their trauma inwards, using strategies such as alcohol misuse to deal with their distress (Liebling-Kalifani 2004).

The medicalization of childhood behaviour and attention deficit hyperactivity disorder

Similar concerns have been expressed regarding the medicalization of some childhood behaviour, especially with the diagnoses of autism, dyslexia, and most controversially attention deficit hyperactivity disorder (ADHD), which is treated with the mood-altering drug Ritalin (methylphenidate).

ADHD is alleged to be fast becoming one of the most overdiagnosed and, some would argue, also the most over-prescribed childhood 'disease' both in the US and in the UK. In the US, the incidence of ADHD ranges between 5 and 10 per cent, depending on the criteria used. In the UK, there was a dramatic rise in diagnosis from some 69,000 children with 'severe ADHD' in 2000 (Best 2001) to 345,000 by 2003, accounting for around 2.5 per cent of British schoolchildren (Timimi 2005). Although there is a huge controversy over what actually constitutes ADHD, the medical profession tends to speak unilaterally about the condition, and diagnostic criteria and treatment are heavily influenced by the US. At the core of clinical diagnosis are assessments of the 'symptoms' of inattention, hyperactivity and impulsiveness (see table 3.3), and the degree to which these impair child and adolescent development.

Inevitably, these core *symptoms* are extremely controversial as they can be argued to be 'normal' facets of childhood and teenage behaviour which, it has been argued, have always been historically present and are culturally produced (Conrad and Schneider 1992; Timimi and Taylor 2004; Timimi 2005). Since conditions such as ADHD are based largely on value judgements rather than physiological symptomatology, they are difficult to define medically, and can end up being manipulated by dominant beliefs, such as having socially desirable children; thus the concept becomes tied to 'normalizing' noncomformist misfit children and rationalizes an already existing motivation within medicine and psychology to control childhood behaviour.

Traditionally, there was a much greater resistance to medicalizing and diagnosing children with psychiatric conditions, partly due to an understandable aversion to prescribing powerful mind-altering drugs to children, but also perhaps due to the deeply entrenched notion of children as emotionally incomplete and incompetent adults who required adequate socialization (Mayall 1996). Victorian ideology into the first half of the twentieth century viewed children as being endowed with strong and dangerous Hobbesian impulses that parents needed to curb to prevent mayhem and destruction, as exemplified in William Golding's *Lord of the Flies* (1954). A paradigm shift after the Second World War, influenced by Rousseau's notion of the child as *tabula rasa* needing education and stimulation, resulted a more innocent vision of childhood (Mayall 1996; James, Jenks and Prout 1998).

However, the process of childhood socialization has been largely concerned with training and controlling bodies and emotions to conform to context-appropriate rules and norms, but the late twentieth-century emphasis on children's rights and on understanding children as a marginalized minority group has resulted in conflicting views:

Table 3.3 Clinical diagnosis of ADHD

Diagnosis label	Criteria	Core signs	Additional diagnostic criteria
ADHD/ADD 1. combined type 2. predominantly inattentive (ADD) 3. predominantly hyperactive/impulsive (ADHD)	DSM IV	Inattention Hyperactivity Impulsivity	1. signs persist for at least 6 months 2. clinically significant impairment in social/academic functioning 3. impairment is present in 2 or more settings (e.g. home & school) 4. signs do not occur during psychotic disorder/other mental disorders
Hyperkinetic disorder	WHO 10	Inattention Hyperactivity Impulsivity	All of above plus all 3 core symptoms present before age 7

Source: Best (2001: 2)

On the one hand, trying to control a child's impulses is viewed as potentially abusive of human rights, on the other [those] impulses are viewed as a danger to society and a threat that has to be controlled. (Timimi 2005: 140)

Children's social worlds mediate between participation in child–adult transactions and their everyday emotionally embodied experience. Mayall (1996) suggests we perceive largely adult models of what children are, how childhood should be lived, and how, since childhood is a relational concept, adults should behave in relation to children. These understandings differ according to setting and, variously, they structure the way homes, schools, health and welfare agencies operate. Most crucially, because of the authority and control adults exercise over all aspects of children's lives, adult models importantly affect children's experience, knowledge and identity; they are critical in constructing the personhood of children (Hockey and James 1993). The requirement that children be happy can lead adults to protect them from knowledge that might sadden them, such as the death of a relative, or the cruelty people enact towards each other. Girls learn not to develop their muscles, if they are to be socially acceptable; and to restrict their bodily movements within smaller spaces than boys do (Young 1990). Children, more perhaps than any other social group, are required to control and organize their emotions (emotion work) and to use these controls to organize bodily movement in ways approved by their superiors and by more general social legitimation.

Children literally learn to manage their bodies at school through emotional control as although school in the UK encourages high valuation of bodily skills in specified times and places, generally children subordinate bodies to minds in a formal regime. They have to sit still, form orderly queues, ask permission to go the lavatory, to eat, drink and exercise at adult-specified times and places. Whilst children may be in tune with their bodily needs, they may not be able to satisfy them, for adult agendas and authority prevent this. Five-year-olds pointed forcibly to adult controls over their bodily management; notably, by the age of nine children had carried out the emotion work necessary to accept these controls and sometimes to circumvent them. The price some of them pay is boredom. (Bendelow and Mayall 2000)

Relationships between adult and child groups, and how close their interests are, in other words 'generational proximity', is defined by Mayall as:

> a continuum ranging from conflict to harmony in child–adult relations. At one extreme, the generations may be experienced as separate, firm, congealed, and standing face-to-face or in opposition to each other, to the extent that the child feels controlled, excluded or defined as object. At the other extreme, children and adults may be engaged in a joint enterprise, in harmony, with similar goals, and with a mutual emotional reinforcement of their satisfaction with the enterprise and the social relationships embedded in it and strengthened through it. (Mayall 1996: 138)

Generational proximity concerns how far the separation or intersection of the two groups, children and adults, allows children to participate in constructing the social order, and we are arguing here that intersections of these two sets of factors are critical in structuring children's experience and in conditioning their agency. This is because children, uniquely compared to other social groups, are positioned as socially, economically and politically dependent on another social group – namely on adults. At school, children's experiences reveal sharp social separation between children's and adults' interests in contrast to the more individually and intimately focused parent–child interaction experienced by most (although not all) children in their homes.

Up until the 1990s, if intervention was required, emotional and behavioural problems in children were largely explained and treated psychodynamically. In this way, developmental psychology and the so-called *psy* disciplines have always performed regulatory roles, and have contributed to the shaping of dominant ideals about 'normal' childhood (Rose 1998), but Timimi argues that the increasing bio-medicalization of childhood behaviour illustrates a growing 'moral panic' about the problematic behaviour of boys, in particular, who do not conform to dominant cultural ideals, and that the popularity of the ADHD diagnosis:

> mirrors certain cultural dynamics that have resulted in the diagnosis being ideally placed to be used (or rather misused)

to respond to the growing cultural anxiety about children and their development. (Timimi 2005: ix)

ADHD is medicalized through a wide range of professionals, through educators, social workers, psychologists as well as medical practitioners including paediatricians and psychiatrists. However, it is legitimized by assumptions of biological and/or genetic causes implicit in the medical model, with the broader context being considered only as a trigger or modifier of the disease process.

Timimi claims that if there is a 'real' increase in ADHD-type behaviour the causes must be social and environmental (2005: 139) and that claims of scientific evidence for the existence of a biological 'brain' disorder is highly debatable; thus ADHD and associated syndromes are best understood as cultural interventions rather than medical conditions. Social constructionist perspectives have argued for some time that the syndrome is *pseudomedical* and is no more a disease than is 'excitability' (Breggin 2001) and the reductionist approach of the medical model has been heavily criticized for its neglect of social context in characterizing hyperactivity, although these critiques have, until recently, remained largely outside the mainstream of medical practice (Conrad and Schneider 1992: 160).

Medicalization occurs in differing degrees, and is orchestrated by the relationship between professionals, depending on whether challenging definitions of the problem exist (Malacrida 2004). First, there may be problems at the level of conceptual analysis as there are difficulties with the diagnostic criteria and multifaceted interpretations of behaviour (e.g. inattention, hyperactivity and impulsiveness can be due to a variety of factors, including boredom and frustration). Secondly, a 'frame analysis' approach as pioneered by Goffman would indicate that it is possible that, in the case of ADHD, children may well live up to the role they are labelled with, behaving as expected of them, and that their behaviour may be socially negotiated by interested adult parties. Both children and parents may become aware of the benefits and advantages of such labelling and explore its limitations knowing they will be exonerated as they are already stigmatized by having a medical condition.

Although boys outnumber girls with the diagnosis with a preponderance of 4:1, this gender distribution is rarely considered in the scientific literature and research. In contemporary western life, families generally produce fewer children but it can be argued that highly competitive materialistic societies have raised expectations for children to succeed in modern life, especially in the field of educational attainment, and it is certainly the case in the UK that boys are less likely to achieve educational success than girls, and this is exacerbated when analysed by class as well as gender (but is far less clearcut in relation to ethnicity). Alongside socioeconomic arguments, explanations for this phenomenon range from blaming the breakdown of the nuclear family and the rise in single parenthood, with subsequent lack of fathers as role models, to cultural critiques of masculinities, to educational practices, but the commonly held popular assumption that boys are genetically pre-programmed to misbehave does not appear in the research literature.

However, it has also been argued that the 'rebiologization' of anxiety and depression in the 1990s has given rise to optimism about the possible treatment of previously intractable behavioural disorders. Medically defining these problems, rather than stigmatizing or even criminalizing them, may bring new understandings of the social processes involved in the development of and response to medical diagnosis and treatment, including a critical framework to analyse medicine and health. Furthermore, medically defining a problem can provide an enormous sense of relief to parents who at best may be extremely frustrated by being unable to understand the behaviour of their child, and at worst may feel an overwhelming sense of failure and individual guilt and blame. Similarly the burden of highly disruptive activity in classrooms on teachers who are under enormous pressure with curriculum targets and league tables may be alleviated by medical intervention, even in the form of medication, rather than having to resort to extreme measures such as exclusion from class. Thus thousands of parents and teachers plus, to a less known extent, children themselves, have embraced the diagnosis and treatment with relief in preference to being excluded from school, or worse.

Disease mongering

The growing tendency to consign young people who do not conform to a chronic illness trajectory with its associated drug regime of Ritalin and similar pharmaceutical treatments (discussed in detail in the next chapter) is simultaneously a grave cause for concern and an important part of the growing deconstructionist critique of contemporary patterns of medicating a wide range of conditions and disorders, known colloquially as *disease mongering*, a term which is gaining widespread use in the medical as well as the social scientific literature. Another example, much discussed in the media, is the increasing numbers of drugs being used to treat a range of syndromes under the rubric of *sexual dysfunction*. Again, behavioural therapies were the traditional interventions for the wide range of associated difficulties including relationship problems, infidelity, depression, performance anxiety, fear of failure and loss of attraction. More recently, pharmaceutical quick-fix solutions for 'unsatisfying sexual performance' are promised with drugs like Viagra, but their development has been heavily criticized as another example of unnecessary medicalization (www.newviewcampaign.org). Leonore Tiefer, a New York academic and convenor of the Campaign for a New View of Women's Sexual Problems, maintains that the creation and promotion of female sexual dysfunction is a textbook case of *disease mongering*:

> [It is] a process that encourages the conversion of socially created anxiety into medical diagnoses suitable for drug treatment. People fed a myth that sex is natural, at the same time as expecting high levels of performance and enduring pleasure, are likely to look for simple solutions. The pharmaceutical industry has taken an aggressive interest in sex to create a sense of sexual inadequacy and interest in drug treatments. The public finds medicalization attractive because the notion of simple scientific solutions fits in with a general overinvestment in biological explanations. (Tiefer 2006)

As in the cases of PTSD and ADHD, sexual dysfunction is yet another example of an increasing range of conditions which may have been previously classified as disorders of behaviour and emotion but which have now become highly, and some would say inappropriately, medicalized.

Emotional health: enlightenment or overmedicalization?

In chapter 1, a paradigm shift from biomedical to integrated models of healthcare (table 1.3) was advocated to encompass more social and holistic understandings of illness and disease, and to address the reductionism of Cartesian dualism. Understanding health and illness along a spectrum rather than polarized notions of being either ill or healthy allows for emotional health and wellbeing to be considered in tandem with physical symptomatology. However, the status of distress and suffering as 'illness' is highly contested, as we have seen, and some critics would claim that much of what are termed disorders of emotion and/or behaviour in Busfield's distinction (1996, see figure 3.1) are not 'real' illnesses to be treated by medicine.

The balance between offering help and intervention to those suffering severe and disabling distress, and the overmedicalization of behaviour or emotions which may respond to more traditional and less dependent coping strategies is an uneasy one. As Hochschild points out, emotional distress is yet another aspect of modern life which tends to be 'outsourced' rather than dealt with internally:

> the counsel of parents, grandparents, aunts and uncles, ministers, priests and rabbis holds relatively less weight than it would a century ago, that of professional therapists, television talk show hosts, radio commentators and agony aunts assume relatively more weight. (Hochschild 2005: 82)

The pharmascepticism and anti-medicalization lobbies claim that the rebiologization of so many disorders and conditions and the increasing use of drug therapies, abetted by media and drug company promotion, have raised public expectations of fast cures so high that dependence on pharmaceutical solutions and associated dissatisfaction rates have rocketed. In his insightful anti-totalitarian novel published in 1932, Aldous Huxley predicted the socially engineered society of *Brave New World* which largely depended on the drug 'soma' to chemically regulate and eliminate unhappiness, dissatisfaction, protest and nonconformity. Some critics fear that trends in contemporary society indicate Huxley's vision may be far from fictional; in the next chapter we consider further the pitfalls of the medicalization of emotional distress, and the 'quick-fix culture'.

4
Medical Responses to Emotional and Psychological Distress

Key concepts: pharmaceutical industry, biological treatments, iatrogenesis, SSRI controversies, talking cures, psychosocial intervention

The medicalization of emotional distress

Chapter 3 charted the limits of the divisions between mental and physical diagnoses of illness, through a range of medically defined disorders and conditions. Although the concept of emotional health can be employed to address the mind/body divide and has enabled destigmatization of 'mental disorders' (at least those which are not associated with psychosis or 'dangerousness') to some extent, it still tends to be the case that illnesses without clear and demonstrable scientific physiopathology remain at the bottom of the hierarchy. Across the whole range of medical care and practice, psychiatry and psychiatric treatments have always been, and still are, subject to huge controversy, carry less prestige and receive less funding for research.

This chapter charts how therapeutic responses to clinically diagnosed mental illnesses emerged over the course of the twentieth century, and focuses in particular on the controversies about the medicalization of emotional distress and anti-social behaviour through mood-altering drugs.

As Rogers and Pilgrim point out (2005), the manifestation of emotional distress is endemic across all cultures, although interpretation and responses may vary widely. Across most of 'western' society, madness and emotional instability have always aroused public response and intervention, and the growth of scientific medicine in general and psychiatry in particular has meant that medicalization has been the most dominant means of response since the nineteenth century (Foucault 1973; Porter 2002). Although psychoanalysis enjoyed a particularly significant influence in psychiatric practice up until the 1940s, which resonates still through the growth of talking cures and counselling, the development of biological and neuro-psychiatry has largely dominated therapeutic responses to emotional distress across the spectrum from severe psychotic mental illnesses to the range of neurotic anxiety and depressive disorders discussed in the last chapter. It is no small irony that most of what is termed *mental illness* has largely been treated with physical or biological interventions, including psychosurgery and electroconvulsive therapy, but most dominantly pharmaceuticals, as illustrated by the following case study.

Case study: Maureen

Maureen was born just before the start of the Second World War, but was apparently not much affected by the experience during her childhood in a small industrial town in North Yorkshire. Her mother came from a large family of shopkeepers, who all lived near each other, and her father worked as a crane driver for a steelworks on his return from the army. Maureen had a younger brother, but was often described as being like a 'spoilt only child', a very pretty girl but reported by her mother to be 'very demanding and selfish'. She trained at secretarial college and was married at 19 to Alfred, an ambitious and upwardly mobile young man who worked as a transport clerk in a nearby town. Shortly after the birth of their first daughter, in 1955, he accepted a post in Kenya as an administrator in the process of handing over the colony, beset by the political turmoil of the Mau-Mau independence movement. Although the couple had never travelled outside England before, and despite the British exodus at that time, the family settled into the newly independent republic, living a privileged and colourful life in post-colonial 1960s Nairobi society.

After giving birth to a second daughter and a son, Maureen worked full-time as PA to the director of an American pharmaceutical company. Freedom from child-care and domestic labour was supplied by reliable, loyal but underpaid workers, as inherited through colonial tradition. Despite the glamour of a seemingly idyllic life, the marriage hit difficulties when, aged 28, she began an affair with her boss. At the same time, she started to take daily doses of codeine tablets (available without prescription), which she claimed she was taking to relieve tension headaches. Over the next few years, her husband claimed her addiction worsened, and she became extremely emotionally volatile, often causing scenes in the diplomatic circles her husband socialized in, which caused him great hurt and embarrassment.

One Sunday, when alone in the house with her younger daughter, aged 11, Maureen took a potentially fatal overdose, but was discovered by the child in a delirious state, sobbing that her lover had ended the affair and that she no longer wanted to live. The daughter managed to telephone for help and Maureen was rushed to hospital. She survived a stomach pump, although was thought to have some kidney damage. Two further attempts over the next few years, and the lack of psychiatric services, prompted her husband to eventually leave Kenya and return to Yorkshire in 1970 in the hope of getting some treatment for her.

Alfred was appointed as an HR director to a firm in York, bought a house in an attractive part of town and ensured the children, now in their teens, and trying to accommodate to a different culture and lifestyle, attended the local grammar schools. Maureen saw a psychiatrist regularly, the codeine was replaced by pre-scribed antidepressants (amitriptyline) and she was able to work at a nearby factory as a secretary for a while. In 1972 she had a severe breakdown, when she was admitted under the Mental Health Act to a private mental hospital. She was diagnosed with psychotic depression and forcibly administered psychotropic medication by injection and ECT on admission.

From this point on, Maureen was in and out of mental hospitals for the rest of her life, and was more or less continuously taking daily medication, a cocktail of anti-depressants, tranquillizers and hypnotics in various combinations. She gained several stones in weight, was continually tired and lethargic, and did not ever return to work. In the early 1980s, Alfred's post was moved to Stratford-upon-Avon, and the eldest daughter settled nearby with her husband and children, playing an important role in Maureen's care. Although the son initially lived with his parents for a year after leaving university, during another dramatic breakdown, he and the other daughter became increasingly estranged from their parents, and moved to London to pursue their careers, visiting only sporadically.

In the mid 1980s Alfred was made redundant from his Stratford post and took up a job in Saudi Arabia. Maureen joined him, but for the first time in her life began to drink alcohol with other expatriates, and within months was drinking heavily. After nearly two years of living in Saudi, she returned to the UK, staying with her eldest daughter whilst Alfred was away, but her drinking problems exacerbated, putting enormous strain on the young family. She went to London to visit her younger daughter, who also had a new baby, and ended up being admitted to the local A&E, vomiting blood after drinking a bottle and a half of vodka. Although the paramedics warned her daughter she might not survive, she recovered remarkably quickly, and safely detoxified from alcohol whilst in hospital. She also stopped taking psychiatric medication during this time, and for several months claimed to feel better than she had done for many years.

This period of stability was shortlived, as in 1987 she began to exhibit behaviour which eventually was interpreted as classic symptoms of hypomania, including delusions of grandeur, sexual disinhibition and flights of ideas which made her thought processes impossible to follow. She became increasingly vulnerable when she spent time alone in her apartment away from the watchful eye of her exhausted daughter – as well as running up huge credit card bills, she would telephone friends and relatives in the early hours of the morning, inviting them to the 'biggest party in the world', and then go out onto the streets to invite strangers to participate. Eventually Alfred had leave his Saudi job and come home to relieve his daughter of the burden of care, and Maureen was again sectioned into a private mental hospital in Northamptonshire with a diagnosis of severe manic depression (bipolar disorder). She spent the next few years being admitted and readmitted there, unable to spend more than a few months at a time at home despite the familiar heavy medication, which now included lithium, a common treatment for bipolar disorder, known to cause liver and kidney damage, and required constant monitoring by blood tests.

In late 1991, Maureen was yet again admitted voluntarily to the Northampton hospital with severe depressive symptoms. She was also complaining of pain, and investigations revealed urinary tract infection. She was eventually moved to a general hospital near to her home for investigations, as she had become progressively bedridden, claiming to be in constant unbearable pain. Most of the health professionals involved in her care at that time, and indeed her family, dismissed her symptoms and her requests for constant painkillers as symptoms of her mental illness and addictive tendencies. In February 1992, a large tumour was discovered on her right kidney. She died the same day without ever knowing her diagnosis of cancer.

The role of pharmaceuticals in psychiatry

Three historical phases have been outlined in the development of these treatments (Pilgrim 2005). Within psychiatry, medicines were not widely used until the so-called 'pharmacological revolution' of the 1950s with the development of powerful antipsychotic drugs such as Largactil (chlorpromazine), alongside mood stabilizers, minor tranquillizers such as Valium (diazepam) and the early antidepressants. The asylums in the 'pre-revolutionary phase' from the late nineteenth/early twentieth century had already emphasized biological causation of mental disorder and relied heavily on physical treatments of restraint and constraint, seclusion and cold baths, but very few drugs apart from bromides and opiates were available and were inevitably used to aid sedation and control. The biological emphasis could also be seen in the ethically dubious development of technological 'innovations' or, more cynically, experiments in the form of interventions such as narcolepsy (literally keeping patients asleep for long periods), lobotomy (operations on the frontal lobes of the brain) and the infamous electroconvulsive therapy (ECT).

The second phase (Pilgrim 2005) was described as a revolution because the widespread use of psychotropic drugs meant the cessation of much of the overt physical methods of constraint such as locked wards and straitjackets which symbolized and stigmatized the Victorian asylums. These advances in medicine were seen as enlightening and liberating, releasing the asylum from its dreadful images of human zoos, subjecting patients to degradation, cruelty and violence, and very much as part of the march of progress. Psychotropic drugs could control delusions and hallucinations, enabling patients to take part in social rehabilitation programmes, and the innovation of 'depot' injections (antipsychotic medication suspended in oil administered monthly rather than daily oral doses) signalled opportunities for even seriously mentally ill patients to be able to leave hospital.

Between the 1950s and 1970s, doses of antipsychotics and antidepressants became much higher, resulting in accusations of *megadosing* (prescribing unusually high doses) and *polypharmacy*. The large doses and toxic cocktail mixes of psychotropic drugs resulted in severe side effects in chronically mentally ill patients, most noticeably the parkinsonian symptoms of *dystonia* (abnormal muscle tone including neck rotation and eyes turning upward), *tardive dyskinesia* (abnormal muscle movements) and *akathisia* (uncontrollable restlessness), resulting in characteristic shuffling gait, jerky uncontrollable movements and facial tics. In turn, and no doubt unintentionally, this highly embodied and very visually identifiable 'difference' served to intensify rather than to diminish stigma.

Responses to the mentally ill have always maintained an uneasy balance between care and control. The use and misuse of psychiatry as socially controlling and coercive aspects were highlighted by movements such as the anti-psychiatrists and the burgeoning user advocacy groups, and became issues of great public concern in the wider context of civil rights and anti-authoritarianism of the time. Psychiatrists were accused of evasion of responsibility for the iatrogenic consequences of antipsychotics, even blaming patients themselves. The iatrogenic critique was underpinned further by the controversy over ECT, its critics arguing that it is coercive, frightening and causes long-term cognitive deficits, also that informed consent is not necessarily obtained. Similarly it was recognized that psychosurgery, especially the practice of lobotomy, could result in permanent adverse effects such as apathy, epilepsy and intellectual impairment as well as the risks of surgery itself.

Despite the controversies over and unpopularity of biological treatments, it was during this phase (from the 1950s onwards) that the symbiotic relationship between drug companies and the medico-psychiatric establishment was cemented. The iatrogenic backlash against psychotropics in particular prompted the development of 'new' antipsychotics (termed atypical antipsychotics) and antidepressants (the SSRIs – selective serotonin reuptake inhibitors) with fewer side effects. Table 4.1 lists the side effects of the 'new' most commonly used antipsychotics.

Even with a limited understanding of medical terminology, it is clear that there are considerable health risks in long-term use of these powerful drugs, not to mention severe bodily discomfort and demoralization through sensitivity to light, weight gain and sexual dysfunction, and the continuation of the characteristic embodied stigmata of parkinsonian movement and gait, resulting in the clearly identifiable 'community care' label.

Table 4.1 Side effects of 'atypical' (new) antipsychotics

System affected	Side effects
Anticholinergic	Dry mucous membranes; blurred vision; constipation and urinary retention
Cognitive	Sedation; confusion; disturbance in concentration and orientation; symptoms of negativity; worsening of orientation
Neurological	Vary through early, middle and late stages but include akathisia (in 40%), dystonia, dyskinesia, parkinsonism and facial tics
Cardiovascular	Hypertension, tachycardia, ECG changes, rarely arrythmias
Endocrine	Changes in libido, gynaecomastia in males, menstrual irregularities and false-positive pregnancy in females
Gastrointestinal	Increased appetite, weight gain; rarely anorexia, dyspepsia, dysphagia, diarrhoea and vomiting
Genitourinary/sexual	Decreased libido, erectile difficulties, impotence, priapism
Ocular	Lenticular pigmentation, blindness
Hypersensitivity	Agranulocytosis (<0.1%); cholestatic jaundice; photosensitivity and skin reactions
Withdrawal symptoms	*24–48 hours:* nausea, vomiting, gastritis, dizziness, headache, insomnia neurological, i.e. akathisia, dystonia, parkinsonism psychosis

Source: adapted from Zaman and Makhdum (2000)

Social control and 'dangerousness'

The closing down of the old asylums and the ideological shift towards community care (which was rarely and inadequately provided in a material sense in the UK or US under the antiwelfare policies of the Thatcher/Reagan regimes) provided the backdrop for government to collude in promoting pharmaceuticals as a solution for relieving mental distress and disorder in the community (Samson 1995). Defenders of the treatments maintain that the benefits of the drug regimes, such as enabling chronic psychiatric patients to live in the community largely free from persecutory delusions and hallucinations, are justified by the severity of illness, and can be seen to outweigh the physiological risks. More cynically, chronic psychoses, especially in the form of paranoid schizophrenia, form a significant threat in public perceptions of *dangerousness*, requiring psychiatry to act as an agent of social control. This function is retained through the remaining psychiatric units and the use of the Mental Health Act (1953, 1983).

Like many other psychiatric labels, 'dangerous and severe personality disorder' (DSPD) is a highly controversial concept. It refers to those people who are thought to be at risk of violent or aggressive behaviour as a direct result of a personality disorder, typically antisocial personality disorder or borderline personality disorder. The term is therefore used to describe certain individuals who are thought to be 'dangerous', either to themselves or to others, and who lack insight into the social and moral consequences of their actions: in lay terms, these are 'psychopaths' (Scott, Jones, Cane, Bendelow and Fulford 2008), but even those working within the psychiatric services view the diagnosis of DSPD with scepticism as it does not appear in the DSM-IV or ICD-10 classification systems as a mental disorder. There is controversy and uncertainty about whether an individual with DSPD is mentally ill or socially deviant, literally 'mad or bad' (Kendell 2002). DSPD emerged as a new category of behaviour following the high-profile case of Michael Stone, who was convicted of murder shortly after being released from hospital on the grounds that his personality disorder was untreatable. This evoked political debates about risk and dangerousness, as well as ethical debates about whether it was more important to protect individual freedom or public safety. A controversial new Mental Health Bill was drafted in 2002, recommending that 'dangerous' individuals could be detained in hospital against their will, even if they were deemed untreatable, in the interests of protecting the public from crime, and is under debate at the time of writing (Mental Health Act Commission 2007).

Psychiatric treatment in the community

The so-called 'third phase' heralded the trend for mental health problems to be treated in primary care and GPs began to prescribe drugs to treat 'mild to moderate' conditions dominated by anxiety states and depression. Thus, the 1970s and 1980s saw a huge rise in GP prescriptions for minor tranquillizers, antidepressants and sleeping pills, and in turn pharmaceutical companies began to target GPs, laying the foundation for the 'quick-fix' culture with brands such as Valium and Librium. The role of pharmaceutical companies became increasingly controversial over the course of the twentieth century because of the huge increase in their profitability and influence from the 1980s, second only to armaments in the US economy (Abraham 1995).

Whereas on the one hand it is important that the benefits of medicines are realized and increased, it has also been the case that prescription drugs can be detrimental to public health when they are unsafe, ineffective or unnecessary as in the infamous case of thalidomide. In the 1990s in the US, adverse reactions to prescription drugs were the fourth leading cause of death among hospitalized patients, after heart disease, cancer and stroke. Other contemporary and controversial issues include access to medicines at affordable prices in developing countries; the neglect of pharmaceutical research and development on diseases where treatments promise only small markets; the promotion and advertising of medical drugs; the comparison of drug treatment with non-drug therapies or so-called alternative remedies (Abraham 1995).

The testing and approval process is under scrutiny because of alleged unfairness in drug testing and regulation processes which are all too often biased towards the commercial interests of pharmaceutical companies at the expense of public health. Psychiatry has been heavily involved in these controversies with the widespread growth in the medicalization of emotional distress or disorder involving pharmaceuticals (in other words, diagnosis of social behaviours as medical conditions treatable with drugs).

Government regulation requires pharmaceuticals to be tested for safety and efficacy, to prove that they are actually effective in treating the illness for which they are being developed. However, this testing process is controlled and largely conducted by the pharmaceutical company developing the drug. Before the drug can be marketed, data from this testing process must be submitted to government regulatory authorities who are responsible for assessing the safety and efficacy of new drugs before granting marketing approval. Whereas only safe and effective drugs are supposed to be approved for marketing, Abraham (1995) maintains that these and other biases towards commercial interests occur at the expense of the interests of public health because, on the whole, pharmaceutical manufacturers control the entire drug testing process and there is a general tendency to award the benefit of the scientific doubt to the drug. Economically the pharmaceutical industry is extremely important to the government in terms of the balance of payments and employment, which promotes a permissive approach to conflicts of interest by expert advisors to regulatory agencies, and reinforces the secrecy of the testing and regulatory process, aided by the ever-revolving door of regulatory personnel. As a recent *Guardian* article pointed out, in the UK, it costs approximately £500 million to bring a drug to market:

> Because randomised trials are so spectacularily complicated and expensive they are beyond the reach of governments, academia and even small companies: only huge international pharmaceutical corporations can afford to run drug trials now, and so drug companies are in complete control of information. (Goldacre 2007)

Although recent drug scandals (in particular surrounding the painkiller Vioxx and SSRIs such as Seroxat) have exposed the commercial bias of multinational pharmaceutical companies that researchers such as Abraham and Healy have repeatedly highlighted, their economic power and financial dominance of randomized controlled trials appear impossible to challenge.

The SSRI controversies and pharmaskepticism

During the course of the 1990s, the ultimate pharmaceutical 'quick fix' evolved, namely the antidepressant group of drugs known as the SSRIs (selective serotonin reuptake inhibitors). Unlike the old antidepressants such MAOIs (mono-amine oxidase inhibitors) and the tricyclics, which although effective had distressing side effects, these new drugs claimed to be completely free of these (see table 4.2 for the side effects as described in psychiatric texts) and Prozac, Zoloft and Paxil quickly became household names (Healy 2004).

They were also popular because their actions were able to be explained in understandable and destigmatizing terms. Inevitably, explanations of emotional or mental distress which explain symptoms as bodily or chemical imbalances rather than as disorders of mind or thought are more readily embraced. Depression and anxiety are thought to be caused by a lack of serotonin production (which can even be measured by a blood test) so in true biomedical mode a simple pharmaceutical 'cure' is produced by chemical replacement. Furthermore stigma is lessened because the whole process can be likened to 'respectable' medical illnesses such as diabetes, with SSRIs in the role of insulin.

As noted in chapter 3, there are also alarming parallels with Huxley's *Brave New World* (1932), where the drug *soma* is taken by the masses voluntarily to produce mood stability and eliminate unhappiness, but in a more sinister vein, also suppresses individualism and anti-authoritarianism in a deceptively totalitarian and socially engineered society of the future. Of course mind-altering substances have and always will be used, whether clinically prescribed, legally sanctioned or prohibited. Superficially, the *quick fix* may seem very attractive, and there are many people who claim to have experienced great benefit from a short course of SSRIs which may have lifted the misery or quelled the anxiety that was blighting their life and remotivated them to participate fully again. However Healy (2004) points out that whereas antibiotics removed certain diseases completely, SSRIs do not 'cure' depression, but merely provide a short-lived chemical high which does not tackle deep-seated causes of severe emotional distress. Healy and other sceptics maintain that we have entered an Age of Depression despite the existence of these 'happy pills' and that we have to understand the 'biobabble' which has replaced the psychobabble of Freudian terms that so coloured our identities during the twentieth century, almost another language through which we can understand ourselves (Healy 2004).

Moreover, despite the claims of no or minimal side effects (see table 4.2), the prescribing of SSRIs has given rise to hundreds of legal actions following suicides and homicides (for example the *Tobin vs SmithKline* case resulted in a first ever finding against a pharmaceutical company for a psychiatric side effect of a psychotropic drug). In addition, the spectre of dependence hangs over these drugs, with recently filed class action for physical dependence on Paxil/Seroxat. Their advocates, both lay and professional, claim that there

Table 4.2   'Official' side effects of selective serotonin reuptake inhibitors

System affected	Side effects
Gastrointestinal	Abdominal discomfort, nausea, vomiting and diarrhoea (usually early and transient)
Metabolic	Hyponatraemia
Neuropsychiatric	Anxiety, headache, restlessness
Sexual	Lowered libido, orgasmic difficulties
Withdrawal symptoms	*Somatic:* dizziness, incoordination, lethargy, nausea, headache, fever, sweating, insomnia and vivid dreams
	Neuropsychiatric: dyskinesias, paraesthesia, electric-shock-like sensations, anxiety, agitation, irritability, confusion, rarely aggression, impulsivity and hypomania

Source: adapted from Zaman and Makhdum (2000)

may be more risk of suicide with SSRIs but they are less toxic than older antidepressants.

Similar arguments are made for and against the medicalization of childhood disorders and especially the prescribing of the psychostimulant Ritalin (methylphenidate hydrochloride; MPH), which is an amphetamine-like addictive drug which is said to mimic the biochemical properties of cocaine for children diagnosed with ADHD. As we saw in chapter 3, parents and teachers in particular eagerly embraced the ADHD label as a means of coping with children and teenagers perceived to be out of control, whereas previously the only measures were drastic and highly stigmatizing, such as exclusion from school. In the US, Novartis (who produce MPH under the brand name Ritalin) and other drug companies producing similar drugs for use in hyperactivity and attention deficit disorders have been very successful in persuading psychiatrists and health authorities of the alleged benefits, despite the potential risks and contraindications. Proponents assert that MPH works by correcting a 'brain disorder', 'biochemical imbalance' or 'biological dysfunction' but no scientific rationale has proved these claims (*British Medical Journal* 1998).

Although MPH is not licensed for use in children under six, there are claims that it is given to children as young as three and is contraindicated in those who suffer marked anxiety, agitation or tension, or have a history of drug or alcohol dependence as well as a range of physical conditions. There are further claims that MPH actually exacerbates many of the symptoms it claims to relieve, but a NICE report (National Institute for Clinical Excellence 2000) essentially endorsed the use of MPH in the UK, noting the only common side effects as nervousness and sleeplessness. Nevertheless, the use of MPH remains highly controversial, with groups such as the UK Hyperactive Children's Support Group claiming that ADHD is caused by nutritional deficiency and can be remedied as such (Best 2001), and, even more extreme, two lawsuits were filed in the US in 2000 asserting that Novartis and the APA (American Psychiatric Association) conspired to create a market for the compound, alleging:

> Ciba/Novartis planned, conspired and colluded to create, develop and promote the diagnoses of Attention-Deficit

Disorder and Attention-Deficit Hyperactivity Disorder in a highly successful effort to increase the market for its product Ritalin. The APA conspired, colluded and cooperated with the other defendants while taking financial contributions from Ciba as well as other members of the pharmaceutical industry.
(Charatan 2000)

Although the APA furiously refuted that it conspired with others to create the diagnosis for the DSM (trial result), the Ritalin scandal, along with the Prozac and Seroxat cases, continues to fuel the so-called Prozac wars and disease-mongering lobbies.

In the twenty-first century, medicalization is a highly complex process, which has benefits as well as costs, and may be equally and eagerly sought out by the lay population rather than simply being imposed by neglectful or unreflective health professionals. If we accept that some forms of emotional distress or disorder do require intervention, there is a problem in deciding between what is 'real' distress or illness and the process of disease-mongering which leads to overprescribing. These criticisms come from within medicine and psychiatry as well as from social scientists, and are enshrined in the debates and controversies raging in the academic (and to some extent the popular) press through the radical movement known as *pharmaskepticism* (Moncrieff, Hopker and Thomas 2005; Menkes 2006).

Lack of consultation time in GP surgeries and under-resourcing of mental health services underpin the readiness to rely on pharmaceutical solutions as the first and easiest resort. Psychiatrists, perhaps more than any other medical professionals, are criticized for being over-reliant on drug company information to guide practice, as their professional training emphasizes the prescribing of drugs and the pharmaceutical companies are highly enmeshed with their professional development (Abraham 1995; Healy 2004). There are increasing concerns that the data from clinical trials, which is voluntarily contributed by the patients seeking healthcare, has become the property of pharmaceutical companies and that a considerable proportion of the therapeutics literature may be 'ghost written'. Healy (2004) claims that much of the data never sees the light of day and puts those who seek help in a state of legal jeopardy. The debates around drugs such as SSRIs play a central part in a growing set of issues in the world of academic medicine, surrounding academic freedom and the changing face of the scientific literature, and are central to the complex relationship between the medical profession, drug companies, public morality, the state and political economy.

Criticisms of psychoneurotechnology

As neuropsychiatry is the most scientific of orientations within the discipline, it continues to retain its high status, despite the accusations of social control, conspiracy theories and the infamous reputations of ECT and psychosurgery, immortalized for successive generations by Jack Nicholson's performance in the film of Ken Kesey's *One Flew over the Cuckoo's Nest* (Kesey 1960). Although ECT is now much less commonly prescribed, comprehensive studies have shown that it is administered to over half of long-term severely mentally ill psychiatric patients in the UK, estimated to be in excess of 11,000 patients, over a fifth of whom receive the treatment by compulsion (Pilgrim 2005).

However, there appears to be wide variation between trusts within the UK, and in 2003 the National Institute for Clinical Excellence(2003) advised doctors that ECT should only be used in cases where all other treatments have failed. In contemporary mental health care, psychosurgery, which involves cutting or destroying part of brain, has diminished in use and is mainly restricted to obsessive-compulsive disorders (OCD), again only recommended where all other interventions fail.

Because biological approaches to psychiatry assume that mental illness is caused by biological malfunctioning, increasing emphasis is given to funding research into genetic causes, and to developing research and treatment around brain imaging. Advocates of essentialist biological explanations of mental illness claim that this could actually be more humane because it could provide a cure for distressing chronic conditions. Moreover, it is argued that proof of genetic transmission could reduce stigma and underpin civil rights as, if a disorder is shown to have a biological basis, it is unjust and inhumane to exclude and persecute people born this way. Cynics claim that scientific causes have never historically prevented prejudice, as racism, sexism and social exclusion of the disabled have all been based on 'biological' or physical characteristics, and warn of the eugenic dangers of genetic determination.

Similarly, despite the high status and funding of brain imaging, which links psychology, psychiatry and neuroscience in developing new tools for noninvasive imaging of the living brain, the practice raises a host of ethical issues. In addition to the classical bioethics of safety and informed consent (e.g. for scans involving radiation or high magnetic field strengths), the ability to correlate brain activation, psychological states and traits raises new prospects and problems. In addition, brain scans are often viewed as more accurate and objective than in fact they are.

Alternative approaches to biomedicine within psychiatry

Although treatment response in 'western' psychiatry is overwhelmingly medicinal, there always has been eclecticism, and in the UK there is a long history of mental health professionals, including psychiatrists and medically qualified therapists, who work with psychodynamic approaches or 'talking cures'.

The impact of psychoanalysis, and the legacy of Freud and his followers from the end of the nineteenth century, has created an intellectual phenomenon that has impacted in immeasurable ways on contemporary life – as a social theory, a 'science' of the mind, even as a way of reading and interpretation, although international associations may formulate competing orthodoxies. As a form of therapy which originated in 1895, psychoanalysis in its purest form (involving three or four hourly sessions per week) has never been widely available and has largely consisted of private practice restricted to an elite clientele. However, the notion of the *unconscious* and that any intervention into improving the human condition cannot be reduced to a technical elimination of 'disorder' (Holmes 2002), is fundamental to enlightened thinking, and the basic principle that repressing trauma inevitably leads to emotional dysfunction or distress is widely accepted and expressed in everyday parlance as 'bottling things up' or needing to emotionally 'explode' or 'spill out'. The strong notion that good relationships rebuild or enhance mental health underpin the provision and growth of 'talking cures' ranging across psychotherapy, behaviourism, cognitivism, humanism, existentialism and general systems theory. Unlike biological interventions, talking cures are anxiously sought and gratefully received, as illustrated by the exponential growth of counselling services during the latter half of the twentieth century, not only within the primary and secondary healthcare system, but also even more accessibly through schools, universities, voluntary organizations and workplaces (Pilgrim 2005: 99). The overall evidence supports the widely held intuition that benign supportive conversations are helpful to people (Pilgrim 2005), but is less clear *which* interventions are most effective. Drugs are cheaper to deploy than labour-intensive psychotherapeutic interventions, therefore there has traditionally been low investment by the state and the medical profession, and despite the increase in acceptance and popularity of talking cures, psychotherapy is still mainly the preserve of the middle and upper classes and privately funded rather than within the NHS (Pilgrim 2005).

However, since the 1996 NHS Strategic Review *Psychotherapy Services in England* advocated an evidence-based comprehensive provision of psychotherapy, policy developments such as the *Mental Health National Service Framework* (Department of Health 2001a) and the Department of Health's *Treatment Choice in Psychological Therapies and Counselling* (2001b) emphasize that psychological therapies 'can be seen as equal players alongside physical and social measures in the management and prevention of mental illness' (Holmes 2002). Evidence-based guidelines are provided to help health professionals to recommend appropriate therapies for depression, eating disorders, panic disorders, obsessive compulsive disorders and deliberate self-harm. It is also increasingly recognized that psychosocial interventions can reduce the probability of psychotic experiences returning, with claims that relapse rates can be reduced by as much as 50 per cent.

Although many of these recommendations acknowledge the pluralistic and multifaceted aspects of psychotherapy, which manifests through a wide range of treatment options, more often it is cognitive behavioural therapy (CBT) which is the intervention of choice for a whole range of conditions including depression, eating disorders, panic disorder, obsessive compulsive disorder, self-harm and even, more recently, psychosis. CBT is easy to understand and learn, achieves behaviour change in reasonably short-term focused interventions and is often less expensive than prescription drugs, all factors which make it popular with government and funders, as well as the evidence-based claims of its effectiveness (Holmes 2002; Tarrier 2002). However, its critics warn of the dangers of its being yet another quick-fix approach that yields superficial short-term results without addressing the deeper causes (Bolsover 2002: 294).

Ironically, although psychotherapeutic approaches are presented as *the* alternative to biological interventions, they are also open to accusations of social control and *normalization*. Training in psychotherapy, and particularly psychoanalysis, is highly selective and very expensive, and inevitably most therapists in the UK tend to be stereotypically white, highly educated and upper or middle class. Clients have to display an acceptable level of articulation to receive therapy, which may exclude some social groups altogether, and alienate others. Stereotypical assumptions and values of therapists about social class, ethnicity, sexuality and gender have all been cited as barriers to viable therapeutic experience. For instance in the case of gender, there have been charges that many basic psychoanalytic concepts can be interpreted as sexist (Mitchell 1975), so therapists may have diminished expectations for female clients and may foster traditional gender roles (which may also be a problem in homosexual relationships). On the other hand, talking cures have also been accused of addressing women's needs more than men's, in that heterosexual men find emotion sharing more difficult as help seeking is discouraged by masculine gender roles in terms of denying feelings and not expressing vulnerability. Like biological interventions, psychodynamic approaches generally can be criticized for lacking social context.

Social contexts of mental illness

Social models of mental illness usually make distinctions between social constructionism, discussed in some detail in the last chapter, and *social causation*. Social causation explanations of mental illness rely on empirical evidence and adopt a positivistic model, hence are successfully assimilated into psychiatric discourse and research because they accept the legitimacy of biomedical diagnoses and medically defined illness such as depression and schizophrenia but suggest that the aetiology is *social*, rather than biological, and generally is associated with social disadvantage. This model gained credibility in the 1980s when the findings of a highly influential study by Brown and Harris (1978) of working-class mothers indicated that a combination of social factors such as having three children under the age of five years, lack of support from an intimate partner and the death of a mother before age eleven could predispose these women to develop clinical depression. Thus, in this model, mental illness is the result of social, economic and cultural factors, and a wealth of evidence for this viewpoint comes from research that has demonstrated an increased risk of mental illness among people living in poverty.

Statistical evidence can show that children of families in the UK in social class V are approximately three times more likely to have a mental health problem than those in social class I (Mental Health Foundation 2005) and that for both men and women the risk of developing a mental health problem is greater among those in deprived areas. This is replicated across the UK: adults in the poorest one-fifth are twice as likely to be at risk of developing mental illness as those on average incomes (Mental Health Foundation 2005) and people with mental health problems are almost three times more likely to be unemployed than all other disabled people (Smith and Twomey 2002). Furthermore, poverty, unemployment and social isolation are associated with the first incidence and prevalence of schizophrenia; and first admission rates to specialist psychiatric care for people with schizophrenia are higher among those resident in deprived areas (Mental Health Foundation 2005).

However, social causation models also have limitations because, although social and cultural factors may create relative risks for a population or class of people, it is unclear how such factors raise the risk of mental illness for an individual, and the link between social ills and mental illness is more accurately *correlational* rather than causal. Put simply, not everyone growing up in poverty becomes mentally ill and, just as in the critiques of biomedical approaches, the precise causes of most mental disorders are not known.

The implications of social causation models for treatment centre on community care initiatives, but the provision of suitable housing projects which provide the necessary levels of support and care is woefully inadequate and underfunded. This picture seems unlikely to change with the dismantling of welfarism and, although social causation models are accepted as making an important aetiological contribution to the understanding of emotional ill health, the logical 'treatment' pathway, namely to alleviate poverty and to improve social conditions, is regarded as utopian and beyond the remit of medicine and psychiatry, admittedly with some justification.

These pragmatic difficulties mean there is little funded research into 'social solutions' but there are exceptions. For instance, a little-reported WHO study was launched in 1967 to determine whether the diagnosis of schizophrenia exists in all countries and whether it could be reliably diagnosed and treated (Hopper, Harrison, Janca and Sartorius 2007). It was highly ambitious in its scope and tracked 3,300 patients spanning a dozen countries including capitalist and communist, eastern and western, northern and southern, large and small, rich and poor. The findings not only established that 'schizophrenia' occurs everywhere but, more controversially, argued that patients in poor nations had better outcomes. The study revealed that patients in poorer countries spent fewer days in hospitals, were more likely to be employed and were more socially connected. Between half and two-thirds became symptom-free, whereas only about a third of patients from rich countries recovered to the same degree. Nigerian, Colombian and Indian patients also seemed less likely to suffer relapses and had longer periods of health between relapses. Doctors in poorer countries stopped drugs when patients became better – whereas doctors in rich countries often required patients to take medication all their lives.

Western psychiatrists were so shocked by the initial findings in the 1970s that they assumed something was wrong with the study and repeated it, but it yielded the same result. The best explanation, researchers concluded, is that the stronger family ties in poorer countries have a profound impact on recovery, which prompted the following memorable quote from Professor Saraceno, the WHO Director of Mental Health at the time:

> If you have a cardiovascular problem, I would prefer to be a citizen in Los Angeles than in India. If I had cancer, I would prefer to be treated in New York than in Iran. But if you have schizophrenia, I am not sure I would prefer to be treated in Los Angeles than in India. (Saraceno 2002)

He went on to point out that most people with schizophrenia in India live with their relatives or in other social networks, in sharp contrast to the United States, where there is much more reliance on the medical and public infrastructure and where most patients with schizophrenia are homeless, in group homes or on their own, in psychiatric facilities or in jail. Other factors cited are that many Indian patients are given low-stress jobs by a culture that values social connectedness over productivity; patients in the United States are usually excluded from regular workplaces; and Indian families sit in on doctor–patient discussions because families are considered central to the problem and the solution.

Thus the implications of the study are that better prognoses can be attributed to the social involvement of extended families and primary care workers to constantly monitor patients and bump up medication dosage at the earliest sign of a psychotic flare-up, whereas nuclear families in more urbanized societies are often unable to provide that kind of help and monitoring. Advocates of the study suggest that the key to treating schizophrenia lies in integrating cultural and social supports with medicine:

> The astounding result calls into question one of the central tenets of modern psychiatry: that a 'brain disease' such as schizophrenia is best treated by hospitals, drugs and biomedical interventions. Anti-psychotic drugs that help quell the outward symptoms may actually exacerbate social withdrawal – drugs cannot replace social supports. Treating schizophrenia without anti-psychotic drugs is unthinkable in the current system in wealthy countries which merely brings patients who are in crisis into hospitals, stabilizes them with drugs and discharges them after a few days – the familiar 'revolving door'. (Saraceno 2002)

Despite these apparently ground-breaking results, the WHO study is rarely quoted in the psychiatric or scientific literature.

Values-based medicine and post-psychiatry

Post-psychiatry has been heralded as another major challenge to the biomedical model, providing a pragmatic and viable new direction for mental health (Bracken and Thomas 2006). Although the movement builds upon the conceptual frameworks of anti-psychiatry, practitioners of post-psychiatry begin by accepting that emotional or mental distress is 'real' in the sense that clinical intervention is needed to alleviate the often severe problems experienced by individuals. They also accept that psychiatry is the dominant mode of dealing with distress, however limited diagnoses and treatments may be. They engage with the principles of VBM which begin with the premise that values affect every stage of the clinical encounter, and, by accepting and working with the diversity of values, opportunities arise for discussion, consultation and negotiation. In other words, the medical model is used as the basis of providing intervention, but diagnosis and treatment are negotiated with the client/user/sufferer (terminology may vary but 'patient' is less likely to be used).

Building on the ethical reasoning approach of VBM outlined in chapter 1, this approach emphasizes the significance of social, political and cultural contexts for the understanding of mental illness and draws attention to the importance of values, rather than causes, in research and practice, giving rise to a so-called 'new philosophy of psychiatry' (Fulford, Dickenson and Murray 2002). Whilst recognizing the importance of empirical knowledge, it gives priority to interpretation and to meaningful experiences. It argues that mental health practice does not need to be based on an individualistic framework centred on medical diagnosis and treatment. User movements argue the need for an open, genuine and democratic debate about mental health, and Bracken and Thomas (2001, 2006) suggest that post-psychiatry is the post-modern deconstruction of modernist psychiatry. If modernist psychiatry is made up of three elements (technical reasoning and a belief in science; exploration of the individual self; and coercion and control of madness), Bracken and Thomas assert that this agenda is no longer tenable because of various postmodern challenges to its basis. These include questioning simple notions of progress and scientific expertise. The rise of the user movement, with its challenging of the biomedical model of mental illness, is seen as being of particular importance. Recent government policy emphases on social exclusion and partnership in health are viewed as an opportunity for a new deal between professionals and service users.

Post-psychiatry proposes a new relationship between society and madness and challenges doctors to rethink their role and responsibilities, building on critiques of antipsychiatry and 'failures' of community care. For example, in relation to the proposals for reform of the Mental Health Act, decontextualizing the biomedical model weakens the argument for relative medical control of the detention process. So post-psychiatry provides a challenge because of emphasis on lay experience and agency, and promotes 'democratization'.

Integration in medical interventions for emotional distress/disorder

Although medicalized responses to emotional distress have acknowledged pluralistic approaches such as talking cures and psychosocial interventions, biological treatments (particularly in the form of pharmaceuticals) have dominated the field of psychiatry and emotional health, and continue to do so with the renewed emphasis on seeking biological and genetic causes. However, the limitations of this biomedical response are subject to enormous controversy in the form of *pharmaskepticism*, namely this dominant tendency to rely on pharmaceutical or technical interventions for simplistic solutions to highly complex illness syndromes.

As this book has highlighted, the precise causes of many contemporary illnesses, especially those involving mental disorders or emotional distress, are unable to be pinpointed, and there is an increasing emphasis to acknowledge that the broad forces that shape individual responses are synergistic. It therefore follows that the causes of health and disease generally can and should be viewed as a product of the *interplay* or *interaction* between biological, psychological and sociocultural factors. This is not just the case for mental health, but can be applied to all areas of health and illness. For instance, diabetes and schizophrenia alike are viewed as the result of interactions between biological, psychological and sociocultural influences. In some cases, a biological predisposition is necessary but not sufficient to explain their occurrence, whereas for others, a psychological or sociocultural cause may be necessary, but again not sufficient. Subsequently, this integrated approach needs to be adopted in modes of treatment, as well as in diagnosis. The next chapter examines the role of complementary and alternative therapies in attempting to bridge the mind/body divide.

5

Complementary Medicine and Alternative Healing Systems

Key concepts: CAM, complementary medicine, alternative/ holistic healing systems, integrative medicine

The medical acronym CAM

Complementary or alternative medicine (CAM) is the generic term encompassing the vast number of systems and practices of healthcare, which for a variety of cultural, social, economic or scientific reasons have not been adopted by conventional biomedicine (otherwise defined as scientific, allopathic or 'western' medicine). Folk medicine, herbal remedies and 'lay' healing practices have existed since antiquity, and alternative healing systems have continued to proliferate even with the advent of biomedicine. Terms applied to therapies not commonly included in mainstream medicine have repeatedly changed over time, evolving historically from the negative *quackery*, the cynical terms *questionable*, *unproven* through *unorthodox*, *unconventional* and *alternative*, and more positively to the use of the term *integrative medicine*. It has been argued that the growth in popularity of these therapies has emerged in response to the decline of faith in biomedicine during the second half of the twentieth century (Cant and Sharma

1999), and moreover that the accelerated proliferation of therapists and clients since the end of the 1980s has been an important factor in challenging biomedical power (Williams, Gabe and Calnan 2000). As we saw in chapter 1, the practices subsumed under the acronym of CAM are extremely wide and diverse, including psychological treatment and support, nutritional approaches and herbal remedies, massage and relaxation techniques, psychic and faith healing as well as the range of alternative healing systems such as Ayurvedism, traditional Chinese medicine (TCM), homeopathy and naturopathy.

Mind/body approaches to healing

Aakster (1986) proposes a form of classification based on distinctions between ancient and modern, sacred and secular (see figure 5.1).

Acupuncture, acupressure and reflexology, for instance, all share the idea of energy meridians running through the body. Under normal circumstances, in a healthy person, the life force *chi* flows evenly, maintaining balance between the vigorous yang and the restraining yin elements. However, if either yang or yin becomes too dominant, bodily harmony is jeopardized and illness may result.

	SACRED	**SECULAR**
ANCIENT	Faith healing Prayer Meditation	Acupuncture Shiatsu Herbalism
MODERN	Christian Science Spiritualism 'New age' religions	Osteopathy Homeopathy Aromatherapy

Figure 5.1 Holistic healing systems (derived from Aakster 1986).

Alternative approaches: the example of cancer

In western scientific medicine, cancer is defined as the uncontrolled or malignant growth of cells that have failed to maintain the normal cellular cycle of creation, growth and death. Thus, the primary aim of conventional cancer treatments, such as chemotherapy, radiation and surgery, is to stop the malignant process by interfering with the growth and spread of such cells. The key goal is that of *cure* which is defined as the absence of detectable signs or symptoms of malignancy for five years from the date of diagnosis.

Some healing practices, in particular those that originate from non-western cultural traditions, may approach cancer from a distinctly different perspective. It is not always possible to use a western evidence-based approach and some of these treatments are unable to be evaluated in a scientific manner. For example, in traditional Chinese medicine the concept of cancer as a disease process may not exist and western terminology may be essentially irrelevant. Instead, a 'cancer' patient is treated according to the tenets and methods of the practice, which aim to support the patient's innate ability to heal, as TCM views people as ecosystems in miniature. Any imbalance between opposing forces, such as yin–yang, heat–cold, dampness–dryness, or disruption in the circulation of *chi* or *qi*, meaning life energy or vital force, produces illness. Maintaining the balance and the flow of 'life elements', therefore, is essential to the maintenance or restoration of health. Treatment is then geared to correcting imbalances or disruptions, possibly with herbal formulas or acupuncture.

Likewise, the ancient healing techniques of Ayurvedic medicine are based on the classification of people into one of three predominant body types. There are specific remedies for disease, and regimens to promote health, for each body type. This healing system has a strong mind–body component, stressing the need to keep consciousness in balance, using techniques such as yoga and meditation and emphasizing regular detoxification and cleansing through all bodily orifices. Similarily, homeopathy and naturopathy, although having their own philosophies and treatments, rely on the belief that the body will repair itself and recover from illness spontaneously once a healthy internal environment is achieved. All these approaches seek to optimize the body's natural ability to eliminate any unwanted growth or invasion, as do the many herbal remedies including mistletoe, saw palmetto, black cohosh, bromelain, curcumin, milk thistle, phytoestrogens, quercetin, rosemary and Saint John's wort.

Many of these remedies are being evaluated in an evidence-based manner through scientific trials, but have not yet been 'proven' to halt disease progression. As they may also interfere with conventional treatments, many medical practitioners view them with suspicion or even hostility. Less contentious and widely used complementary treatments are nutritional supplements (including acidophilus, antioxidants, calcium D-glucarate, coenzyme Q10, DHEA, fish oils, folic acid, ginseng, melatonin, pyridoxine and vitamins B6, B12 and D) and dietary measures (green tea, fibre, soy, garlic, onion, fruit and vegetable consumption have all been strongly associated with protective effects against cancer).

However, in line with the turn to holism, recent advances in medical treatment have led to the development of newer cancer treatments that aim to exploit the patient's natural capacity to eliminate the malignant process by boosting the body's immune response. Other therapies which oncological research includes under the CAM rubric are psychological treatments and supports (including psychotherapy, imagery, group therapy and cancer support groups), and massage and relaxation techniques such as aromatherapy and psychic healing (prayer, laying on of hands).

CAM usage in cancer

In the late 1990s, a systematic review across 13 countries indicated that CAM usage in cancer ranged between 7 per cent and 64 per cent with an average prevalence of 31 per cent (Ernst and Cassileth 1998). Subsequently, the International Union Against Cancer (UICC), an international, non-government volunteer organization, e-mailed a questionnaire concerning alternative therapy use to its members, receiving responses from 33 different countries (Cassileth, Schraub, Robinson and Vickers 2001). Descriptive analyses of this dataset were conducted, indicating the existence of a large and heterogeneous group of unproved remedies used to treat cancer in both developed and developing countries around the world. Market research surveys (e.g. Datamonitor 2006) indicate that up to 80 per cent of cancer patients used an alternative or complementary modality.

It seems to be clear that, notwithstanding the methodological difficulties of defining alternative therapies, large numbers of cancer sufferers have adopted non-biomedical treatments and Cassileth (1999) emphasizes that 'the absence of consistent results across studies is due primarily to differing definitions of unconventional cancer therapies from study to study. Cancer patients are always looking for new hope, and many have turned to nontraditional means.'

A considerable amount of more detailed survey research has been undertaken since the millennium, with estimates of CAM usage in cancer ranging between 40 per cent and 80 per cent. Richardson, Sanders and Palmer (2000) assessed the prevalence and predictors of CAM use in 453 attenders of the University of Texas Cancer Centre, Houston. Overall 99 per cent of the sample had heard of CAM and 83 per cent had used at least one CAM approach. Use was greatest for spiritual practices (80 per cent), vitamins and herbs (63 per cent), and movement and physical therapies (59 per cent), and predicted by sex (female), younger age, indigent pay status, and surgery. After excluding spiritual practices and psychotherapy, 96 per cent of participants were aware of CAM and 69 per cent of those had used CAM. Claims that the interest in CAM use in cancer patients has grown dramatically were made by Bernstein and Grasso's study (2001) of 100 adult cancer patients in a private non-profit South Florida hospital who completed a descriptive cross-sectional survey questionnaire. The mean age of participants was 59 years; 42 patients were male and 58 female. According to the survey results, 80 per cent of patients reported using some type of CAM; 81 per cent took vitamins, 54 per cent took herbal products, 30 per cent used relaxation techniques, 20 per cent received massages and 10 per cent used home remedies. Among patients who took vitamins, 65 per cent said they took a multivitamin, 39 per cent took vitamin C and 31 per cent vitamin E. The most common herbal remedies used were green tea, echinacea, shark cartilage, grape seed extract and milk thistle. Meditation and deep breathing were the two most common relaxation techniques practised. A large majority of cancer patients are using CAM. The researchers recommended that in the light of the growing interest in CAM, healthcare professionals need to be educated about the most common therapies used.

Similar patterns of CAM usage across the developed world have been recorded: a large national survey in Australia (Adams, Sibbritt and Easthope 2003) revealed that 30 per cent of cancer patients attending various clinics (n = 319) reported that they were using alternative therapy (the most frequently given reasons were a preference for natural therapy, and seeing the alternative therapy as another source of hope). Dietary and psychological methods were most prevalent, followed by herbalism. Seventy-five per cent of patients tried more than one therapy. 83 per cent used at least one CAM approach. Use was greatest for spiritual practices (80 per cent), vitamins and herbs (63 per cent), and movement and physical therapies (59 per cent). Another Australian study of breast cancer patients (Salminen et al. 2004) reported an even higher take-up of CAM (39%), whereas a study in China revealed lower rates of CAM take-up than in the US. Abdullah, Lau and Chow (2003) found usage of CAM in 352 breast cancer patients in China to be 28 per cent whereas, in Japan, a survey of 192 hospitalized cancer patients in the National Shikoku Cancer Center showed 32 per cent using CAM (mainly dietary supplements with a small minority using acupuncture). All studies again confirmed the majority of users as young to middle-aged, female, having higher education and having used allopathic treatments conjunctively. Similarly, in the UK, a recent study revealed that although 32 per cent of patients in an oncology clinic in Southampton were receiving some form of CAM (the most popular were massage, nutrition, aromatherapy, relaxation and homeopathy), 99 per cent would very much have liked to have access to these treatments (Lewith, Broomfield and Prescott 2002).

Social characteristics of CAM users in cancer: who uses it and why?

Generally, studies reveal that cancer patients who seek CAM therapies tend to be better educated, of higher socioeconomic status, female, and younger than those who do not (under 50). Typically, they are more health-conscious and utilize more mainstream medical services than do people who do not use CAM. Although socio-economic classification (SEC) is seen to be a factor, the issue of access to CAMs (namely whether these treatments are supplied free within the healthcare system or whether they have to be paid for) is rarely explored in these studies.

Given that breast cancer disproportionately affects those of higher socioeconomic status and that sufferers are almost exclusively female, it is not surprising that estimates of CAM usage are higher than in both the general population and in other forms of cancer. For example, Di Gianni, Garber and Winer (2002) estimate CAM use among their sample of women with breast cancer, at 42 per cent, to be higher than among individuals in the general population (most popular were nutritional/dietary supplements, relaxation strategies and social support groups) and claim that usage is also strongly correlated with psychosocial distress. Another recent study of 551 women with breast cancer who had already received conventional treatments (Henderson and Donatelle 2004) showed an even higher rate of CAM take-up, with two-thirds using at least one therapy (most popular were relaxation/meditation, herbs, spiritual healing and megavitamins). The reasons given were to enhance quality of life, to feel more in control, to strengthen the immune system and to reduce stress.

As well as the gender and social class dimensions, there may also be ethnic and cultural factors which exacerbate the need to clarify which treatments are being used; Richardson, Sanders, Palmer et al. (2000) studied the types and prevalence of conventional and alternative therapies used by women in four ethnic groups (Latino, white, black and Chinese) diagnosed with breast cancer from 1990 through 1992 in San Francisco, and explored factors influencing the choices of their therapies. About half of the women used at least one type of alternative therapy, and about one-third used two types; most therapies were used for a duration of less than 6 months. Both the alternative therapies used and factors influencing the choice of therapy varied by ethnicity. Blacks most often used spiritual healing (36 per cent), Chinese most often used herbal remedies (22 per cent) and Latino women most often used dietary therapies (30 per cent) and spiritual healing (26 per cent). Among whites, 35 per cent used dietary methods and 21 per cent used physical methods such as massage and acupuncture. In general, women who had a higher educational level or income, were of younger age, had private insurance, and exercised or attended support groups were more likely to use alternative therapies. Other studies have confirmed little variation across ethnic groups in overall use of CAM, but show diversity in preferred therapies (Kakai et al. 2003; Mackenzie et al. 2003).

Complementary therapies have often not been tested using conventional scientific methods, so their effects have not been measured or proven. Although there may be scant scientific evidence that these therapies halt disease progression, the small amount of qualitative research undertaken with cancer patients using CAMs reveals a range of carefully thought-out reasons and motives, namely that they want to explore all possibilities, to feel more in control and more hopeful, and to help manage the deep emotional distress of the experience of cancer (di Gianni et al. 2002; Adams et al. 2003; van der Weg and Streuli 2003). The deeply metaphorical and frightening nature of cancer itself (Sontag 1978), the depersonalizing aspects of scientific medicine and invasive side effects of radiotherapy and chemotherapy make treatments which focus on the interaction of mind/body/spirit and quality of life very attractive. Although there is scarce qualitative research in this area, recent studies indicate that, on the whole, cancer sufferers use a mixture of conventional and alternative treatments, the main reason being to enhance wellbeing, with a tiny minority holding 'unrealistic' expectations of cure (Lewith et al. 2002; Henderson and Donatelle 2004).

The use of complementary therapies in chronic pain: experiences from the DipEx project

Another area of medicine in which complementary approaches have an increasingly important role is in chronic pain and pain management, in which some therapies are becoming increasingly 'mainstream'.

The DipEx project features in-depth interviews with people suffering with chronic pain and found that on the whole they tended to be broad-minded about approaches to managing pain, with a consensus that different approaches work for different individuals, even if attributed to a 'pseudo' or placebo effect. Interviewees stressed the importance of getting as much information as possible about complementary approaches from a range of sources (GPs, the Internet and support groups) and put much emphasis on choosing a therapist who was registered and personally recommended.

Some, although not all, interviewees felt that it was important to keep their GP informed of different things they were trying in case they were perceived as unsuitable or adversely affecting the traditional treatments they were using. A wide range of therapies had been tried, including homeopathy, chiropractic, osteopathy, reflexology, acupuncture, massage, herbal medicines, spiritual healing and reiki: sometimes a whole range by just one person as in the following account.

Case study

Aromatherapy massage, yes, I love it and I'd love to go every week, twice a week, but I just can't do it. It's too pricey. It's £30 to £35 for an hour's full massage. There's no point in just going for a leg massage or a neck and shoulder massage when you've got fibromyalgia because it affects more or less all your body. So yes, I'd love to see something like that, that you can go to your GP's surgery and get at least once a week, but it's pricey. If you can afford it, do it, because it is wonderful. It's something I would do on a regular basis if I could afford it but it's just not affordable and I go as and when I can. I've tried shiatsu which made my muscles even more painful. I've tried reiki, three sessions of that and I didn't feel I was getting anywhere. At £40 a session it's a lot of money, I think. Some of the alternative therapies, while I think they could be quite good, some of them can take a wee while to work and you really need to have a fair amount of money that you want to spend because they are not cheap. I consulted a herbalist who made up a potion for me. £35 consultation fee for an hour. Very good, took all my medical history and various things like that. Made up a potion for me which cost about £18 I think which lasts for 3 weeks. After 3 weeks you go back for a follow-up consultation, that was £20, and then you had your potion again which was changed slightly I think the second and third time, again you had that to pay for so it works out quite pricey and to be honest I didn't, well I probably slightly alleviated my symptoms, it didn't feel worth what I was paying for.

I also tried Chinese herbal medicine. Spent about £300 on that and again I don't feel, a really, slight, very, very slight improvement but not what I would say was really worth paying for. A couple of things that I haven't tried. I've tried things that you can buy out of homeopathic chemists, but I haven't actually spoken to a registered qualified homeopathic person to get any of their remedies. I have heard they can be helpful and then I've heard from other people they're not. I suppose it may be something to think about for the future. And then I've also heard as well you can actually get a referral to a homeopathic doctor on the NHS. I haven't actually queried that with my own GP yet but I've heard it can be done. And I think the other thing which can be quite helpful and that's another thing I'm going to ask my GP about, acupuncture I believe can. But it has to be not something you go for just once or twice like you maybe would with sciatica and things like that. It's something you've got to sort of get on a regular basis so again unless you could afford to pay privately you'd hope you'd maybe get something on the NHS. If you find something and it works and you can find the money to pay for it then you know, stick with it, but anybody can set themselves up as doing alternative therapies so be careful about who you consult. But I would be quite happy to pay for, I'd be quite happy to find the money and pay for some kind of alternative therapy if I knew I was going to get more out of it than anything else but so far, no, I haven't actually found that. Me, personally, I haven't, whether other people have I don't know, but I certainly haven't to any degree which is unfortunate but at least I have tried. I'm open to ideas.

Experiences of each of these therapies yielded a range of opinions: some said they had benefited enormously whereas others had not, but there was much discussion about differing approaches. Massage and aromatherapy were valued because they enhanced sensations of wellbeing, resulting in perceptions of better pain management. Others said that massage helped them to relax and avoid muscular spasms, but only if they were able to trust that the therapist would not hurt them. In contrast, some of the people who were interviewed were very protective of their bodies and could not countenance the thought of deep massage, manipulations, or having their feet or hands touched. There was also some scepticism about complementary therapists: one woman suggested, 'they never say don't come back'. However, this had not been everyone's experience: some people had entered into longstanding 'maintenance' treatment with their therapists, but several others were told that they were unsuitable for acupuncture, or reassured to hear that an improvement should be evident after their first three osteopathic treatments. Others had decided to avoid complementary approaches and preferred to use traditional approaches or pain management techniques.

Dietary approaches and supplements were widely used, but there was some scepticism about consulting professionals:

> I've tried various complementary therapies over the last few years . . . I got a book written by a nutritionist and I read up on all the various vitamins, minerals, amino acids, and everything a body should be taking, you know I've tried out various

vitamins, changed my diet, not 100 per cent but I've changed a good 75 per cent of my diet in that I don't really drink tea, coffee, don't eat white bread, tend to eat more brown bread. (DipEx interview CP12)

Those who knew that their diets were inadequate, or affected by problems such as irritable bowel syndrome, felt that vitamin and mineral supplements were a wise precaution whereas others said supplements were expensive and unnecessary:

I eat my five portions of fruit and veg every day. I eat oily fish, don't like it but I eat it, I eat, I try to sort of eat all the things that are good for you that are healthy. I've tried various different kinds of vitamins, minerals, amino acids, and usually for a period of two or three months at a time, but to be perfectly honest with you I don't really feel an awful lot of difference with the vitamins and things like that. I think that if you're eating relatively well the things you should be eating, it more or less balances things out for you. (DipEx interview CP12)

Acupuncture had been used by several people in the sample, the most common experiences were of noticeable effects, often not permanent, although some found prolonged pain relief. But by far the most commonly used complementary therapies were chiropractic and osteopathy, and some spoke of 'wonderful' therapists who they trusted to treat their backs, necks and headaches:

I do get quite a lot of bad headaches actually and I tend to find, when I go to him, he puts the vertebrae back sort of, it sounds like there's a crack, it's not painful at all, it sounds horrible when he's doing it, but it's very good and the headache will go virtually straight away. It's absolutely fantastic. So I'm all for saying to people 'Look, you know, well I know somebody that can help you' because the GPs are very good at giving out anti-inflammatories, but that isn't always the answer. Not everybody wants to pop pills and, in fact, tonight I start a college course in reflexology, because I think alternative and complementary medicine is getting quite popular because I think people do want that. They don't necessarily want to pop a pill because it doesn't always work, 'cos that doesn't work with me. So if I think, you know, if he can do that then that's brilliant from everybody's point of view isn't it? (DipEx interview CP20)

Concern was expressed about the potential for unscrupulous private therapists to exploit those who are desperate and vulnerable because of their pain. The following extract from a woman who has had pain for 22 years illustrates the complexities of the process:

> I think anyone with a chronic condition is going to probably consider using complementary therapies at some stage. It is problematical because there is no sort of protocol you can follow as to what you should try and who you should try it with and patients are very vulnerable because they may be told by somebody they know or respect or who's trying to support them. So it becomes a sort of a situation where you ricochet to one therapy and if it doesn't work for you ricochet to another one and there's no rhyme or reason to it, or you can spend an awful lot of money and that's even if you have good therapists and unfortunately it's often very difficult to know who are good, reliable therapists unless you are prepared to do quite a lot of research. There are some ways of finding out using professional registers for people like acupuncturists for instance, or chiropractors, but you have to be quite a knowledgeable and dedicated patient to sort of find out all that information and of course at the very worst you become, you may find yourself in the hands of someone who is a complete charlatan or who actually does you damage in the very worst scenario. So it is very problematical and although personally I think it is worth trying things, I think you should do your research, try to go into it with realistic hopes and try not to be too disappointed if it doesn't work for you. (DipEx interview CP07)

The growth in popularity of CAM

It is clear is that the popularity of CAMs can be seen to have accelerated markedly since the 1990s in Northern Europe, the US and Australasia. Patterns of usage in Southern and Eastern Europe are less clear, perhaps because of the strict regulation of health practitioners in the southern EU states such as Greece, Italy and Spain, where statutory recognition is needed to practise medicine in any form, and this seems to be the case also in Eastern Europe although bans on homeopathy in Hungary, Czechoslovakia and East Germany have been lifted since the fall of communism (Fisher and Ward 1994). Generally it seems that CAM was not encouraged or incorporated into state systems, but not prohibited, acupuncture perhaps being an exception towards the end of regimes; and the liberalization of healthcare systems has led to an upsurge of interest in CAM throughout Eastern Europe. Herbal and folk traditions have persisted throughout, including no doubt in Southern Europe, so CAM usage is likely to reflect the huge increase in popularity revealed by the survey research on CAM usage published in mainstream medical journals.

Eisenberg (1993) estimated that one-third of Americans research and use non-traditional medical alternatives, often without apprising their physicians. A follow-up study in 1998 found that use of at least 1 of 16 alternative therapies during the previous year increased from 39 per cent in 1990 to 42 per cent in 1997. The therapies increasing the most included herbal medicine, massage, megavitamins, self-help groups, folk remedies, energy healing and homeopathy. Ni, Simile and Hardy (2002) claim that the three most commonly used therapies in the US are spiritual healing or prayer (14 per cent), herbal medicine (10 per cent) and chiropractic therapies (8 per cent).

Patterns indicate that general use of CAM in Europe is even more widespread than in the US. Reilly (2001) claims that one in three patients seek 'unorthodox' care and that CAM is the second biggest growth business in Europe with a range of standards from excellent to dangerous. Research in Northern Europe reveals high take-up in Germany, no doubt aided by the *Heilpraktiker* system which licenses practitioners who are not members of recognized health professions to practise provided they have passed an examination in complementary medicine. Tuffs (2002) claims that 75 per cent of the population over 16 have had some experience of CAM and it is generally well established in Germany, apparently in a dialogue with conventional medicine. In their study 41 per cent of patients surveyed were currently receiving some form of complementary medicine and appeared to be more closely involved in the decision process and were more satisfied with treatments than conventionally treated patients.

Complementary therapies in the NHS

The position in the UK has changed markedly since 1994, particularly with the backing of complementary medicine by the British Medical Association in 1993, and surveys over the past decade have reflected a growing demand by the public and interest by health practitioners in reliable, practical and safe natural medicines, especially where conventional treatments are ineffective.

A survey by the BBC claimed one in four people in the UK have tried CAMs and 75 per cent of the public want alternative therapies made available on the NHS (BBC 2007). In addition, it is claimed that 45% of registered medical practitioners refer patients to complementary medical treatments and that 85% of medical students, 76% of GPs and 69% of hospital doctors now feel that complementary therapies should be made available on the NHS. The survey also showed 58% of nurses incorporate or use alternative therapies in their work and 89% recommend alternative therapies to patients. In 1993, a survey conducted by the British Market Research Bureau found that 89% of the population would use complementary medicine (Anon. 1993). GPs have also become more inclined to recommend non-conventional treatments. Dobson (2003) claims that as many as half of general practices in England offer patients some access to CAMs and medical students, doctors and nurses are now actively studying and using CAMs with as many as 70% of hospital doctors and 93% of GPs referring patients to non-conventional health practitioners. In addition, 20% of GPs and 12% of hospital doctors actually practise some form of complementary medicine, and 85% of medical students, 76% of GPs and 69% of hospital doctors now feel that complementary therapies should be made available on the NHS. Overall, it seems that alternative and complementary medicines and therapies are rapidly becoming integrated within GP practices, health centres and hospitals in the UK.

However, funding is a major issue as although some Primary Care Trusts pay for patients to see practitioners, this is relatively unusual. The DipEx project maintains that the biggest deterrent to using complementary therapies is the cost. Almost everyone who had used therapies said that this had been a problem, and for some people who were living on low incomes or benefits it was an absolute barrier, as in this woman's account:

> Once you finish up, you're not getting the wages or the over-time and all that, you're getting a basic, what would you call it incapacity, or whatever they called it at that time, money so you wouldn't worry how much you have or not have, and that's where the support of your family and partner came in financially. You would think, oh I haven't tried it, what is it, oh it's some cream based on this herb or something, so off you go and pay about £19.99 or something for a wee tube and rub it furiously and apply it, and next day you'd wake up and there'd be no cure, and you'd think, oh. And so it went on, I mean I must have spent my family and my partner's money, I think over 2 years or, even say to the present, anything between £2,500 to £3,000, I mean I tried acupuncture, costly, reflexology, costly, aromatherapy, which worked slightly but only for a day, and at that time I think I was paying about £28 for three quarters of an hour in '96. So you tried all these and even to this day when somebody says, 'Oh have you heard of this new thing?' Now you're a bit more wary because you know there is no Holy Grail, because you know you've fallen over so many hurdles because you know, you know, it might not work, you don't really build your hopes up so you try them but you're a bit more careful, I mean if it's £79 you think well, I've had this for 10 years, I'm not going to spend that money on this cure, if it's about £15/£20 or even £30 you think, well I'll give it a shot, but what I'm trying to say is after a number of years and so many false dawns, you're a bit more careful in what you try, especially with the financial limitations.

Homeopathy is unique among all of the alternative and com-plementary therapies as it has been part of Britain's National Health Service since 1948 and is available at five NHS homeopathic hospitals: The Royal London, Glasgow, Liverpool (Mossley Hill), Bristol and Tunbridge Wells. Other therapies can also be made available but largely at the discretion of GP fundholding practices, District Health Authorities (DHAs) or Family Health Service Authorities (FSHAs). In 1992, a national survey carried out among DHAs, FHSAs and GP fundholding practices found that 70 per cent wanted complementary therapies (mostly homeopathy, acupuncture, osteopathy and chiropractic) to be available on the NHS, and 83 per cent of DHAs, although most have incorporated them on an experimental basis (Anon. 1993). Many FHSAs have regarded health promotion clinics as opportunities to employ complementary therapies for smoking cessation, stress management and pain. However, the main barriers restricting the more widespread application of complementary therapies are simply lack of information about the therapies, lack of available evidence relating to their effectiveness, and lack of resources.

According to the national survey report, the single most important factor preventing greater use of complementary therapies into the NHS was the lack of good-quality information on effectiveness and training. However, what is clear is that the process of getting this information to the requisite authorities is slow. What is needed is for the relevant associations and training organizations to become more proactive by marketing their therapies and approaching health authorities and GP fundholding practices. The organizations need to become more involved in research projects, anticipating therapeutic applications that can be evaluated and tested. And, most of all, the relevant organizations need to reverse the trend of fragmented disunity and build national professional bodies working to a common end.

The growth in the use of complementary medicines over the last twenty years in the UK has often been attributed in part to the advocacy of Prince Charles (see, for example, BMA 1993). He has since established the Prince's Foundation for Integrated Health (FIH), which encourages the development of complementary medicines and integrated healthcare. The General Medical Council's position has been clear for some time in that it is open for any family doctor to employ a complementary therapist to offer NHS treatment in his practice provided the doctor retains clinical responsibility and accountability (DoH 1991).

However popular with patients, resistance to NHS provision in the context of widespread NHS cuts in 2006 was voiced by a collective of 13 eminent medics who wrote to *The Times* urging local healthcare trusts to stop backing 'unproven or disproved treatments' like homeopathy and acupuncture and to pay only for medicine 'based on solid evidence'. Their objections centred around two initiatives: a government-funded guide on homeopathy for patients, and the Smallwood report (Smallwood 2005; for comments on Smallwood see Ernst 2006) commissioned by Prince Charles, which suggested greater access to complementary therapies in the NHS might lead to widespread benefits. Homeopathy was described as an 'implausible treatment for which over a dozen systematic reviews have failed to produce convincing evidence of effectiveness', and the letter implied that prescribing complementary therapies through the NHS was irresponsible and wasteful. A spokeswoman for the Department of Health said it was up to clinicians and trusts to decide on the best treatment for a patient.

> We know it is important that as more people turn to these therapies a solid evidence base is developed. Patients rightly expect to have clear information about the range of treatments that are available to them, including complementary therapies. (BBC 2006)

The ensuing controversy rages on to the present, with complementary therapists emphasizing the lack of 'solid evidence' in many allopathic interventions.

CAM: a redundant concept?

Critics from all positions have repeatedly pointed out that CAM covers such an enormous variety of theoretical approaches, therapies and remedies that as an umbrella term it is rendered almost meaningless, thus clarity of definition is crucial to relevant research and investigation.

In addition, most research about the therapeutic benefits of CAM is collected through surveys conducted in clinics, but there is considerable unease and controversy as to whether some of the above therapies are indeed *alternative* or whether they have become integrative to good oncological practice. *Alternative* therapies typically are promoted for use *instead* of mainstream treatment, which may be especially problematic in treating cancer, where delaying conventional treatment may diminish the possibility of remission and cure. Moreover, interventions sold as literal alternatives to chemotherapy, surgery and radiation therapy may be biologically active, potentially harmful and extremely costly. This in turn leads to dismissal and suspicion by medics who view them as unproven methods promoted as alternatives to mainstream cancer treatment, with patients open to financial and emotional exploitation. In contrast, *complementary* therapies are used alongside mainstream cancer care as supportive measures that control symptoms, enhance wellbeing and contribute to overall patient care. There is also an important distinction to be made between remedies which claim to halt disease progression, of which there is very little scientific evidence (Ernst 1999, 2000; Winer 2004) and those which promote wellbeing and healing (Bernstein and Grasso 2001; Ernst, Schmidt and Steuer-Vogt 2003).

Thus treatments promoted as alternatives to mainstream biomedical cures (for example, the recently exposed false 'cancer cure' of Italy's Dr Di Bella; Cassileth 1999) should be distinguished from complementary therapies, which are applied as adjuncts to mainstream care in an integrated fashion. The latter include mind–body techniques and herbal remedies, among many other remedies, all aimed at symptom control and enhanced quality of life, and the term *integrative* medicine is used by many practitioners, and is the preferred term of many acupuncturists, osteopaths, chiropractors and nutritionists working alongside allopathic health professionals in health centres.

Integrated medicine is not simply a synonym for complementary medicine. Complementary medicine refers to treatments that may be used as adjuncts to conventional treatments and are not usually taught in medical schools. Integrated medicine has a larger meaning and mission, its focus being on health and healing rather than disease and treatment. It views patients as whole people with minds and spirits as well as bodies and includes these dimensions into diagnosis and treatment. (Rees and Weil 2001: 119)

This differentiation also provides a clearer understanding of the range and spectrum of therapeutic activity and enables selective evaluation of the clinical and therapeutic effects of complementary and alternative treatments, thus allowing for selective acceptance or rejection.

What is clear is that a broad spectrum of treatments and therapies which are included under the rubric of CAMs, including so-called 'unproven' remedies and treatments, are extremely popular despite the fact that some health professionals may be at best discouraging, if not outrightly hostile to them. However, others may be actively involved in promoting what they see as the beneficial effects which may range from halting disease progression to enhancing wellbeing. Access to therapies thus may vary not only by the preferences of practitioners and patients but also by, at least in the UK, whether they are available on the NHS or privately, and research needs to take account of these cultural and geographical aspects. Fisher and Ward (1994: 109–10) point out national idiosyncrasies, which often relate to national legal situations; for instance reflexology is particularly popular in Denmark because, they claim, acupuncture, to which it is related, is more heavily regulated as it is considered a form of surgery due to puncturing of the skin. Likewise they claim that anthroposophical medicine, inspired by Steiner, is popular in German-speaking countries, the Dutch are keen on spiritual healers, the Finns on massage, and so on.

Understandably clinicians have emphasized the need to ensure that alternative remedies do not have harmful side effects (something that is labelled 'natural' may not necessarily be harmless) and that they do not interfere with conventional treatments. Whereas there is an enormous amount of information available to encourage this 'lay expertise', especially on the Internet, there is the potential for the promotion of alternative remedies to become financially or emotionally exploitative and there is enormous concern over the lack of regulation, which is beginning to be addressed.

However, in the twenty-first century there is recognition that in the process of seeking help and advice from health professionals, people no longer simply do whatever 'doctor says' and that the influence of new technologies and forms of communication, especially the Internet, is radically changing and impacting on doctor–patient and other healthcare relationships between professionals and clients (Marshall and Henwood 2007). Although medical and public opinion may still be deeply divided about the value of non-mainstream therapies, enlightened physicians should surely encourage any measure which enhances physical and emotional wellbeing, with the proviso that both patients *and* doctors obtain safe and accurate information.

6
Holism or Healthism?

Key concepts: health and lifestyle; body maintenance and bodywork: fitness, weight and beauty; healthism and the therapeutic critique; emotional health

Mind/body models: enlightenment or increased surveillance?

This book has focused on trends in contemporary healthcare in the developed world, and particularly within the UK, doubtlessly and implicitly taking for granted the enormous achievements of biomedical science over the twentieth century.

Nevertheless, it is sadly the case that the goals of Nye Bevan at the conception of the National Health Service, namely to deliver healthcare that is accessible, effective, equitable and affordable, largely remains a utopian dream. Alongside the enormous dilemmas of political economy and depleting resources, there are seemingly insoluble problems of faceless, even dehumanizing, aspects of an often overly bureaucratic and burnt-out system, which cannot encompass the complex social and emotional needs of those with chronic illnesses or medically unexplainable but severely distressing symptoms. This book has attempted to chart the shift of focus in models of healthcare in the latter half of the twentieth century, and has suggested that in theoretical rhetoric and, at least in some areas and specialisms, integrated models have superseded biomedical ones to some extent.

A key aspect of this process has been the increasing emphasis on mind–body connections and a rejection of dualistic or monocausal understandings of causes of illness. This is not a polarized argument against biomedicine, indeed the enlightening and healing propensity of science and technology, linked to good evidence-based practice, is obviously fundamental to effective healthcare, but medicine can never be limited solely to science as it is intrinsically connected to human embodiment in all its intricacies.

In her autobiographical account of the embodied experience of a compound fracture of her arm, Ann Oakley eloquently describes the disjuncture between science and subjectivity, the effects of which linger some five years after her accident:

> There is, and remains, this paradox: I don't *feel* normal, although I am, apparently, cured. Classical neurology is based on the concept of function, not on that of 'subjective' perception. Restoration of *function* is what counts, and it's perfectly compatible with a continuing impairment of *sensation*, and of the brain's ability to recognize the repair that's occurred in the damaged limb. This approach fits the body-as-machine model of Western medicine, and the unimportance of what Virginia Woolf called 'the creature within'. It helps to explain why there's been much more research into motor function than into sensibility, despite the fact that, without sensation, the hand is virtually useless. This is why tests of functional ability are a poor guide to what people with damaged hands can actually do. Medical scientists know very little about the relative importance of these two sorts of factors they've identified as important: the peripheral (what happens in the hand) and the central (what happens in the brain). Perhaps the missing link has something to do with the person. (Oakley 2007: 90–1)

In this last chapter, the relationship between the person, the individual and their societal context is pursued further through the mind–body–society connection. In particular, some of the contemporary themes outlined in chapter 1, regarding our bodies as projects to be worked upon and maintained in modern life, are elaborated in order to reflect whether a shift to more holistic concepts of health and illness have facilitated this process through the bodily practices we pursue in the name of 'health'.

It may appear to be axiomatic that the pursuit of 'fitness' and health (including our sexual and emotional health), supported by health education and promotion initiatives, seems a logically enlightened and socially responsible enterprise for any individual. There is even the possibility of widening this model out to mind/body/society as it allows recognition of wider social and political forces outside individual control such as world poverty, war and environmental damage which may or may not engender motivation to organize collectively. Nevertheless the notion that in contemporary society we all have some individual responsibility for own health, albeit mitigated by biological, social, environmental or psychological factors, is becoming ubiquitous. However, the wariness of the so-called 'imperialization' of health in late modernity (Lupton 1995; Williams, Gabe and Calnan 2000; Scambler 2004) has developed into a much more cynical critique of the negative implications of *healthism*, which in turn can be seen to have superseded the notion of medicalization by pervading all aspects of everyday life.

Health and lifestyle

Socioeconomic class has long been linked to health since Edwin Chadwick published his *General Report on the Sanitary Conditions of the Labouring Population of Great Britain* in 1842. This showed that the average lifespan in Liverpool at that time was 35 years for gentry and professionals but only 15 for labourers, mechanics and servants. Although life expectancy has improved for all classes in Britain since this time, inequalities have remained.

The Black Report (Townsend and Davidson 1982) was originally commissioned by the Labour Government in the 1970s, but by the time the report was released in 1980, the Thatcher government tried to suppress the findings which showed that although there had continued to be an improvement in health across all the classes during the first 35 years of the National Health Service, there was still a correlation between social class (as measured by the old Registrar General's scale) and infant mortality rates, life expectancy and inequalities in the use of medical services. The Black Report identified and established four possible explanations for this phenomenon, namely artefact, natural selection, lifestyle and socioeconomic factors (Townsend and Davidson 1980).

Artefact and natural selection explanations have largely been discounted as credible overarching explanations. Although lifestyle and cultural practices were thought to feature significantly in health inequalities, the Black Report and subsequent research (Whitehead 1987; Shaw, Dorling, Gordon and Davey-Smith 1999) consistently point to socioeconomic and material factors as being the main factor in the ever-widening health divide, and include increasingly sophisticated theorizing linking social capital to health. Although correlations between social class and health inequalities continue to be significant (see for instance, National Statistics Socio-Economic Classification (NS-SEC), none of the explanations are meant to be completely monocausal, as they all have limitations, plus the potential to be synergistic (see table 6.1).

Health awareness has become a facet of everyday living, some even term it a 'national obsession' (Furedi 2004; Scambler 2004), and lay perceptions and understandings (including collective enterprises such as politics and the media) play a vital role in defining concepts. The role of health education and health promotion in reinforcing the role of lifestyle choices in health maintenance reaches far beyond government policy and into the popular media, and, some would argue, brainwashes the social psyche despite the lack of research evidence implicating lifestyle as a major cause of illness. For example, a recent study of Australian GPs showed clear distinctions between lifestyle as *cause* of disease or as *risk factor*, in conjunction with other medical frameworks, e.g. biochemical models, germ theories, genetic and psychological explanations, but rarely as the sole cause (Hanson and Easthope 2006: 5). Nevertheless, lifestyle choices have been the main target for governmental health campaigns, since the late

Table 6.1 Limitations to individual explanations of health inequalities

Explanation	Limitations
Artefact	This argument is undermined by the fact that inequalities have been demonstrated using a number of different systems of measurement of social class. These include occupation, property ownership, educational status and access to social resources
Natural or social selection	There is some evidence of 'social drift', where people with poor health suffer a decline in socioeconomic position, but the opposite hypothesis, that the healthy rise in class, is less likely as many health problems only emerge in adulthood, once career choices have been made
Lifestyle/cultural explanations	The 'hard' version of this explanation, that the freely made choices of individuals in each class are responsible for differing health outcomes, is overly simplistic. But there is evidence that risk behaviours are unevenly distributed between the classes and that this contributes to the health gradient
Socio/material and social capital explanation	Poverty is demonstrably bad for health and is the most dominant and scientifically upheld explanation of health inequalities, yet material explanations are not sufficient on their own to explain class differences in health. While life expectancy is lower in poorer, less developed countries, some diseases are more prevalent in the richer West. But when we look at how these diseases are distributed within the wealthy nations we find that they are most prevalent in their poorest regions. The idea that social isolation is bad for health is also supported by self-report studies of social groups excluded from employment

Source: adapted from Wilkinson (2005)

1980s from the publication of *Health of the Nation* (DoH 1991b) onwards, and many of these initiatives, such as the smoking ban and focus on obesity by New Labour, have been welcomed by health professionals and general public alike, as increasing public responsibility and awareness. Other initiatives linked to health in its social context, such as recycling waste and addressing climate change, have developed the collective consciousness to a level which seemed unattainable even a decade ago, when they were often dismissed as 'cranky' 'new age' trends.

Health promotion and the case of sexual health

The end of the twentieth century brought dramatic changes in understanding of human sexuality and sexual behaviour. Although not the only factor, undoubtedly the pandemic of human immunodeficiency virus (HIV) played a major role. The toll taken on people's health by other sexually transmitted infections (STIs), unwanted pregnancies, unsafe abortion, infertility, gender-based violence, sexual dysfunction, and discrimination on the basis of sexual orientation has been amply documented and highlighted in national and international studies (see www.worldsexology.org/).

In line with the recognition of the extent of these problems, there have been huge advances in knowledge about sexual function and sexual behaviour, and their relationship to other aspects of health, such as mental health and general health, wellbeing and maturation. These advances, together with the development of new contraceptive technologies, medications for sexual dysfunction, and more holistic approaches to the provision of family planning and other reproductive health-care services, have required health providers, managers and researchers to redefine their approaches to human sexuality. The sexual health movement promotes an entitlement to 'responsible, safe and satisfying sexual lives' in which sexual (and reproductive) health and wellbeing are essential factors. In this model, sexual health is an essential component of general health and includes the avoidance of unintended pregnancies and sexually transmitted infections. Unintended pregnancies are associated with increased risk of poor social, economic and health outcomes for mother and child, and important sequelae of sexually transmitted infections include pelvic inflammatory disease and infertility, cervical cancer, and increased susceptibility to HIV infection. For some of these factors teenagers are at greater risk than older age groups.

Sexual health requires a positive approach to human sexuality and an understanding of the complex factors that shape human sexual behaviour. These factors affect whether the expression of sexuality leads to sexual health and wellbeing or to sexual behaviours that put people at risk or make them vulnerable to sexual and reproductive ill health. Health programme managers, policy makers and care providers need to understand and promote the potentially positive role sexuality can play in people's lives and to build health services that can promote sexually healthy societies.

Sexual health was defined as part of reproductive health in the Programme of Action of the International Conference on Population and Development (ICPD) in 1994 and included the concept of sexual health as something 'enriching' and that 'enhance[s] personality, communication and love'. It went further by stating that 'fundamental to this concept are the right to sexual information and the right to pleasure'. In response to the changing environment, global organizations such as the World Health Organization work in collaboration with other organizations such as the World Association for Sexology (WAS) to reflect on the state of sexual health globally and define the areas where WHO and its partners could provide guidance to national health managers, policy makers and care providers on how better to address sexual health (www.worldsexology.org/).

Resisting the cult of individualism: mind/body/society contexts

Although holistic models purport to embrace the mind/body/society link, much remains to be done to understand the connections between the environment and illness in contemporary medical models and practices as well as in the explanatory power of science. Health needs to be studied at the nexus between cultural practices, biological activities, social contexts and medical models, which are all deeply embedded within social structures. Furthermore, a sophisticated understanding of how human health links to the environment has important implications for access to healthcare services, for the choice and range of treatments available and for the sorts of interventions undertaken by healthcare practitioners, policy makers, governmental agencies and health activists (Conrad and Jacobson 2003). The traditional sociological rejection of the biological can no longer be sustained with contemporary concerns of global warming and environmental destruction, and Gislason emphasizes the need for medical sociologists to tackle the thorny and complex issues surrounding the biosocial model of health:

> The need to make visible the biological and systems-based aspects of human health and to work across the biology/ sociology disciplinary divides and between the dualisms (such as nature/culture, body/mind, self/other and human/animal) that underpin much of Western thought. (Gislason 2007)

She also points out the tendency for research in health and illness, medical knowledge and healthcare practices to focus on the short-term risks rather than the long-term impacts of prevention; thus seemingly 'objective' biomedical evidence is likely to address distinct components of the disease cycle but is less likely to play a central role in producing integrated knowledge about the relationship between disease risks and the health impacts of prevention programmes.

However, for some critics, recent public health initiatives directed at individual lifestyle behaviours have taken on a much more sinister tone, and 'think tank' lobbies have accused New Labour of buying into the ideologies of the 'Nanny State', namely policies which replace welfare provision with heavy-handed interventions from government, as in this editorial attack on the then Minister for Health:

> Jowell has championed what she refers to as the 'new politics of behaviour', which preaches that government must intervene to save the disgusting, obese, tobacco-raddled, binge-drinking masses from themselves ... Jowell became the first

leading politician openly to champion the concept of the nanny state, although she said she preferred to call it the 'enabling state'. We have long thought it more accurate today to talk about Jowell and Co presiding over a therapeutic state, with the public cast in the role of helpless, vulnerable patients on the couch. (Furedi 2006)

If health is completely individualized in terms of responsibility, there may be subsequent drastic consequences for healthcare delivery, as in the recent example of some health chiefs in NHS trusts in the UK deciding to refuse certain kinds of non-urgent surgery to smokers – including hip and knee replacements. Both trusts were in financial crisis and justified their decision on the basis that smokers are estimated to have three times as many complications as non-smokers, and that their cases would be reconsidered if they attended a smoking cessation clinic. These, and an increasing number of similar decisions, rely on a change of policy by the government's National Institute for Clinical Excellence (NICE) which allows health authorities to take patients' lifestyles into account when deciding whether a particular treatment would be effective. This policy could lead to a complete recalculation of waiting lists along strictly utilitarian lines, with younger, fitter patients, who lead the 'right' kind of lifestyle, prioritized over those who might be more expensive to treat.

Opposition to this trend was voiced forcibly by one journalist who nostalgically recalled an earlier era espoused by the microbiologist René Dubos:

> In the words of a wise physician, it is part of the doctor's function to make it possible for his patients to go on doing the pleasant things that are bad for them – smoking too much, eating and drinking too much – without killing themselves any sooner than is necessary. To force people to live in pain till they fall into line should be a cause for national scandal. It is a measure of how browbeaten we have become in matters of health that it is not. (Dubos 1987)

Dubos maintains that whereas it is appropriate and desirable for health professionals to advise measures to improve health, it is unacceptable and against the Hippocratic oath to refuse treatment altogether. Concepts of lifestyle based almost exclusively on individual behaviours and practices considered to be risk factors for disease are inadequate to account for social context and experience of illness. The current emphasis on individual responsibility for health feeds into the more sinister aspects of healthism and supports accusations that holistic approaches to health may actually increase social regulation and governmental surveillance in an unprecedented way by expanding into practically all areas of everyday life (Armstrong 1995; Lupton 1995).

Body maintenance and bodywork: fitness, weight and beauty

Pierre Bourdieu's concept of cultural capital (1984) suggests self-identity is inextricably bound up with consumer culture and has been shown to be manifested through projects of the body (Shilling 2003; Clarke 2008). The twenty-first century fascinations of 'western society', such as the cult of celebrity and the project of 'the body', make identity and lifestyle into pervasive major foci, backed up by media hype, but also by health promotion campaigns which often focus on individual behaviour rather than taking on board the social aspects of these complex processes. Thus, the rise of healthism is underpinned by the medicalization of weight, appearance and fitness, which has negative as well as more positive implications.

The ideal of health is linked with feeling good, a notion of true wellbeing which rests on a notion of harmony between body, soul, mind and emotion, as well as satisfactory relationships with other people and society as a whole (Coward 1989: 43–4). These processes, in turn, link up with more general trends towards the cultivation of the body as a project in consumer culture and the growth of social reflexivity in late modernity. It is here, within this context, that regimes of body maintenance come to the fore, a movement focused on the body as a machine, which needs to be fine-tuned, cared for, reconstructed and carefully presented through such measures as diet, physical exercise and sporting activities, personal health programmes and designer clothing (Shilling

1993: 35). Within consumer culture the body is proclaimed as a vehicle for pleasure (Featherstone 1982: 21) and both men and women see the body as a project worthy of time and effort. Contemporary body projects may be manifested in preoccupation with bodily maintenance and control through diet, 'fitness' and other body modifications such as cosmetic surgery. The pressure to conform to idealized body images which differ in detail by gender – the ideal for women's bodies across classes, cultures and ethnicities is to be slender with European features, and for men's to be muscular and 'worked out' – has developed dramatically as a sign of cultural distinction since the 1960s (Bordo 1997) and subject to ever-increasing pressure from consumerism and the media. Across both genders, weight is not as critical as body shape and proportion, and the preoccupation with body image is endemic in western culture.

Inevitably the quest for unattainable bodily perfection has given rise to a whole new category of body image disorders and there are myriad diseases, disorders and problem conditions involving food, eating and weight, but in everyday conversation, the term 'eating disorders' has come to mean anorexia nervosa, bulimia and binge eating and is strongly associated with women who are seen to be more dissatisfied with body image. Feminist analyses describe this as 'normative discontent' as a result of a misogynistic society which objectifies women's bodies and experiences (Orbach 1986); the prevalence of eating disorders, especially anorexia nervosa, is considerably higher in females than males. Seen as the compulsive pursuit of thinness, anorexia is heavily medicalized, with high incidences of severe illness and fatalities. Psychosocial explanations for its cause include a moral reaction to gluttony with subsequent stigmatization of fatness, and a fear of pregnancy or of maturing into womanhood (Bruch 1978). Anorexia classically affects young middle-class women and indeed body image disorder is strongly class-related in that socially and economically advantaged women appear to be more dissatisfied than other groups (McLaren and Kuh 2004).

The gendering of eating and body disorders as exclusively female is also being refuted by researchers of male disorders. Phillips and Castle (2001) challenge claims that females are more affected by negative body images and suggest that potentially as many men as women may suffer in this respect, but that the manifestation of this distress may differ. The clinically diagnosed condition known as *body dysmorphic disorder* leads to high incidences of dysfunction in men, ranging from being housebound to hospital admissions and suicide. The condition involves preoccupation with skin, hair, nose or genitals, with repetitive time-consuming behaviours to examine, fix or hide defects such as mirror-checking, comparisons with other men, camouflaging, reassurance seeking, or excessive grooming. Another condition, *muscle dysmorphia* involving compulsive working out and preoccupation with diet, is found almost exclusively in males, as is the abuse of anabolic steroids (Phillips and Castle 2001: 323).These disorders, along with the perennial problems of binge drinking, substance abuse and obesity, militate against the ideals of the 'body as project', and individual shortcomings in attaining socially acceptable bodies may inevitably increase the propensity for disappointment and human misery.

Healthism and the therapeutic critique

Within this context, health now becomes a goal to be endlessly pursued if rarely achieved, and it has become inextricably linked with individual attitudes, commitment and personal responsibility. Perfect health involves self-transformation, 'not just of our bodies and our minds but even of our emotions' (Coward 1989: 46). Over the last decade or so, a movement often termed the 'therapeutic critique' has combined critiques of healthism with those of disease mongering and pharmaskepticism already discussed in chapters 3 and 4. It takes as its starting point that if we accept we are living in a 'risk' society (Beck 1992) as characterized by the fragmentation of social networks and communities and the *atomization* of the individual (i.e. the isolation of individuals within homogeneous social groups), there are implications for emotional health. In his insightful book *The Importance of Disappointment*, Craib described a process of:

cultural pressures, often normal pressures which have to do with wanting to help people, to ease suffering, to be effective, to be good at our jobs, make us vulnerable to the denial of necessity and inevitability of certain forms of human suffering. We set out to cure and we construct blueprints of what people ought to be feeling, ought to be like, and we can too easily set about trying to manipulate or even force people into these blueprints. (Craib 1994: 8)

The phenomenon of the quick-fix culture has been raised earlier, namely the idiomatic term for the tendency to rely on medical interventions, especially in the form of pharmaceuticals, to banish discomfort and distress, indeed any negative experience in addition to pain and illness. Lyon (1996) aptly terms this rapidly growing propensity in modern society *cosmetic psychopharmacology* and she expresses concern as to the inclusion of dysthymia and its vagueness as a diagnostic criterion, resulting in the seemingly endless expansion of the boundaries of clinical depression. Inevitably, she claims, the solution to this dysfunctionality is medicinal, further resulting in 'chemically assisted selves' (Lyon 1996). Despite increased life expectancy and relative material wellbeing, the so-called 'happiness gap' can thus be characterized as a chemical reaction to the difference between the dreams we are sold and the daily reality of life in an advanced capitalist society.

The following passage from Jonathan Franzen's novel *The Corrections* vividly illustrates the obsessional extremes of how, under the twin pressures of high achievement and time, emotional health becomes personal responsibility and lifestyle choice:

Gary was able to understand and track his neurochemistry (and he was a vice president at Cen Trust Bank, not a shrink, let's remember) his leading indicators all seemed rather healthy. Although in general Gary applauded the modern trend toward individual self-management of retirement funds, long distance calling plans and private schooling options, he was less than thrilled to be given responsibility for his own personal brain chemistry, especially when certain people in his life, notably his father, refused to take any such responsibility. But Gary was nothing if not conscientious. As he entered the darkroom, he estimated that his levels of Neurofactor 3 (i.e. serotonin:

a very, very important factor) were posting seven-day or even thirty-day highs, that his Factor 2 and Factor 7 levels were likewise outperforming expectations, and that his Factor 1 had rebounded from an early morning slump related to the glass of Armagnac he'd drunk at bedtime. He had a spring in his step, an agreeable awareness of his above-average height and his late-summer suntan. His resentment of his wife Caroline was moderate and self-contained. Declines led key advances in key indices of paranoia (eg persistent suspicion that Caroline and his two older sons were mocking him) and his seasonally adjusted assessment of life's futility and brevity was consistent with the overall robustness of his mental economy. He was not in the least bit clinically depressed. (Franzen 2002: 159–60).

There is certainly a popular argument that the socioeconomic improvements of life in the western world have meant that, on the one hand, most of us never experience severe hunger or poverty, droughts or extreme climate conditions or infectious diseases that kill, but that the explosion of depression, anxiety, substance misuse and eating disorders is a socially constructed luxury of a spoiled narcissistic society obsessed by material envy, body image, celebrity and reality TV. The concept of *affluenza* or 'luxury fever' has been enthusiastically adopted by the broadsheet media as a portmanteau word to describe this paradox in quasi-medical terms as a middle-class 'virus' brought on by the social and material envy of a society obsessed by:

> flash holidays, luxury furniture, big salaries and expensive cars . . . individualism replaced by consumerism as the aspirational middle classes shackle themselves to unfulfilling jobs, working excessively long hours and cutting themselves off from proper relationships. (James 2007)

The term is thought to have been popularized in the United States in a 1997 documentary from which John de Graaf, the producer, also co-authored a book with the same title, defined thus:

> *affluenza*, n. a painful, contagious, socially transmitted condition of overload, debt, anxiety and waste resulting from the

dogged pursuit of more. 1. The bloated, sluggish and unful-
filled feeling that results from efforts to keep up with the
Joneses. 2. An epidemic of stress, overwork, waste and indebt-
edness caused by dogged pursuit of the American Dream.
3. An unsustainable addiction to economic growth. (ref to
come)

Critics of individualism and consumerism such as Furedi
(2004) have indicated a growing tendency for social problems
to be interpreted as emotional, and for the highly individualized idiom of therapeutic discourse to be used to make sense
of social isolation, through discourses of being 'stressed out',
'burnt out' or having a mid-life crisis. In this model, the use
of personal inadequacies, guilt feelings, conflicts and neuroses
to replace abstract, almost invisible social influences such as
globalization, market forces, cultural and political institutions
is a source of great concern to some contemporary writers
reflecting on 'modern life'. Furedi (2004) has railed against
the tendency for 'social and cultural influence to be discounted
in favour of narrow psychological contemplation'. He con-
tends that the emphasis on achievement of personal happiness
and fulfilment through self-discovery, self-assessment and
self-actualization has resulted in self-esteem becoming *the*
important explanatory variable. In turn, low self-esteem
becomes an overarching explanation for socially perceived
'problem' groups such as teenagers, the unemployed, elderly,
mentally ill, lone parents or the disabled. Furthermore, the
avoidance of negative emotion (because to feel dissatisfied,
disillusioned or miserable is seen as 'unhealthy' or 'pathological') is all too readily absorbed into the post-Thatcher/Rea-
ganite culture of 1980s individualism and, he argues, is *not*
an enlightened shift (Furedi 2004: 23).

Emotional health, integrated models and the need for balance

Integrated models of health and illness are increasingly permeating contemporary healthcare, and are gaining popularity
and credibility within the mainstream medical literature and
research, as the limits of biomedicine become increasingly

evident in contemporary times (Wade and Halligan 2004). Integrated models also challenge traditional sociological assumptions that doctors are only concerned with the biological (disease) and that the social (illness) is of concern outside medicine as 'in everyday clinical practice doctors constantly faced with issues relating to social causes of ill-health and the social contexts of ill-health and lifestyle provide doctors with a framework to talk about the social' (Hansen and Easthope 2006).

Many of these challenges are rooted in 'holistic' paradigms – the notion that the functioning of a whole interrelated system can only be understood in terms of its totality (Samson 1999b: 64) – and therefore actively acknowledge the role the health of the environment plays in determining the status of human health. Systems-based medical cosmologies are, from a historical vantage point, also important to western medicine. Holism was the predominant theoretical norm from Ancient Greece to the Enlightenment and thus the medical system operating in Europe during this timeframe was founded on a belief in the relationship between bodily and cosmic order (Samson 1999a: 4). Hippocratic medicine taught that both health and disease are governed by natural laws and reflect the influence exerted on people by the environment and the degree of harmony with the natural world expressed in their daily lives. Accordingly, health was seen as dependent upon a state of equilibrium or homeostasis among the various internal factors which govern the operations of the body and the mind (Dubos 1987). The four humours of the human body corresponded to natural elements (phlegm to water, blood to air, yellow bile to fire and black bile to earth) and health was achieved through a balanced state of unity when the microcosm (the humours of the person) were in harmony with the elements of the world (the cosmos or macrocosm) (Samson 1999a: 4). Disease was a complex 'concatenation of circumstances' rather than the simple direct effect of the environment acting upon a person. Samson emphasizes that the organic cosmology of sixteenth-century Europe produced a medical cosmology that worked with(in) the notion that the Earth was an organism and that self was linked to society through interdependent community-based relations.

Scientific and medical knowledge has advanced significantly in many arenas since the sixteen hundreds and with it the emergence of nuanced insights into arenas of life studied within biology, genetics and infectious disease medicine. What has been lost, however, is the holistic paradigm, within which studying the environmental determinants of health made sense. In contrast to the present day, contestations to the logic of human–environment interdependence would have been out of place in previous medical cosmologies. Recognizing shifts in medical approaches to human–environment interfaces creates a fissure in the seamlessness of dominant biomedical discourses about human pathology and creates the possibility for a re-engagement with holistic paradigms because they establish that environmental determinants of health have been considered within myriad medical models for millennia. That the impact of social and natural environments on human health is a debated and often contested issue today indicates a great deal about the medical cosmology operating in our time. Recent flares in these debates may be in part a response to the contemporary epidemiological leap taking place, marked by the rise in infectious disease epidemics, but may also anticipate a shift in medical and public health approaches to infectious diseases.

Recent sociopolitical (the rise of the risk society), epidemiological (the return of infectious disease epidemics) and ecological (the visible material impacts of global climate change) shifts are precipitating a conceptual and practical reorganization of medical ideologies and practices. It seems that the notion of interconnection (an element of holism) may be emerging, which can be expressed in epidemiological and social terms: 'by the end of the twentieth century, it was clear that economic globalization had dramatically increased the worldwide epidemiological *"web of interconnectedness"*' (Freund, McGuire and Podhurst 2003: 26). It seems that today within medicine and particularly public health medicine, the Enlightenment view of nature as 'given' is becoming increasingly problematical. Some literature on complementary and alternative medicine suggests that the rise in interest in alternative medicine is a reflection of people's increasing interest in being treated as biopsychosocial beings who are attempting to cultivate more harmony in their own lives and between themselves and their lived (social and biological) environments (see for instance Pietroni 1992; Samson 1999a, b).

Samson (1999b) points out that residues of Hippocratic concepts of health and disease exist within medical practice specifically and within society more generally as 'a medical system that is both environmental and psychosomatic. It is open to the possibility that the state of the body is influenced by natural phenomena, external and internal to the person . . . [and] also suggests that frames of mind and psychological states profoundly affect the body' (1999b: 64). Certainly, the concept of *balance*, which is intrinsically holistic and based on the Hippocratic view of the body as a microcosm of Nature, is crucial to the process of intellectual and conceptual thinking, as it is in understanding and constructing models of healthcare. The dissolution of the artificial divides between mental and physical health is an essential part of this *rapprochement*, and understanding emotions with their propensity to link 'private troubles and public issues' (Wright Mills 1959) is crucial to developing a mind-body-society perspective.

Thus psychosocial overdeterminism in understanding health and illness is potentially as dangerous and as reductionist as biological supremacy.

Bearing the therapeutic critique in mind, in particular as regards the warning that 'Society is much more comfortable dealing with poverty as a mental health problem rather than a social issue' (Furedi 2004: 27), it is essential not to overplay this factor in the equation to the exclusion of all others, and to achieve conceptual, political and practical balance.

Emotion management certainly has the capacity to be used as a form of social engineering, and in this way if emotional dysfunction (i.e. unprocessed and unmanaged emotions) is depicted as a cause of social breakdown, emotional health could be appropriated to impose new conformities, encouraging powerlessness, dependency and the development of the kind of 'sick' society Illich predicted. On the other hand, the concept of emotional health implies destigmatization, accessibility and holistic links between mind, body and even society. As in the discourse of sexual health, the term emotional health is gaining common parlance and is used unproblematically in GP surgeries and on information websites underwritten by proclamations such as 'anyone can suffer mental distress, you are not alone' and 'people talk about aches and pains easily but not about stress and depression' (see figure 6.1).

There appears to be widespread acceptance of the notion that all higher mammals seem to show signs of sadness under conditions of loss or learned helplessness, and that in humans, these feelings are shaped by language (Pilgrim 2005). In turn, the suppression and 'bottling up' of traumatic experience leads to emotional problems, so, inevitably, emotional distress creates health problems and may lead to medically defined illness.

Thus the concept of emotional health is surely an enlightening and desirable one. Furthermore it seems axiomatic that the development of our emotional literacy will ultimately equip us with a more communicative, empathetic and open society, which has far-reaching collective, as well as individualized, implications. Health is such an important variable in social processes, and whether relating to individuals or social groups, it can interact with other characteristics such as gender, race or class to exert a major influence on life chance or experience. Moreover holistic concepts of health enable radical change in what is meant by health, illness and disease, with our sights much higher than simply the avoidance of illness.

Biomedicine may dominate healthcare practice, but it is not the only story as holistic and integrated concepts of health

In this section

Looking after your state of mind is as important as taking care of your body, yet most of us manage our physical health far better than our emotional health.

❚ Wellbeing
Accentuate the positive and appreciate your worth
❚ Stress
Spot when stress is becoming unmanageable
❚ Young people
Adjusting to the changes of adolescence

❚ Phobias and panic attacks
When you have no idea why you're scared...
❚ Self-harming
Self-harm is a way of dealing with strong emotions

❚ Suicidal feelings
There are people who can help you get through
❚ Bereavement
Each person's experience of grief is unique

Figure 6.1   Emotional health. Source: www.bbc.co.uk/health

and illness continue to emanate from within medicine as well as from without. Since the 1970s, the US physician Lynch's illluminating and humanistic work on the role of emotion in medical practice (1977, 1985) has warned the medical profession of the potentially serious implications which stem from the separation of reason and feeling, not only for medical practice, but for human culture in general. Instead of the hopes of a new and better world, designed to end ignorance and superstition, that Descartes envisaged would be based on reason, the ultimate implications of rationality can be seen in a more sinister light:

> It was an idea that at first sparked off great hope and optimism in the West. Yet it was also a blind hope which was crushed forever in the madness of the sheer rationality of Auschwitz, where the mathematical idea of a final solution bore witness to a terrible flaw in the philosophical foundations of modern Western civilization. For it was there, in one of the most sophisticated of all Western nations, that men who were clearly rational were also clearly incapable of hearing the cries of human suffering. If Germany was the most scientific – that is, rational – of all nations, and if it had the most advanced medicine in the Western world, it was nevertheless a medicine almost totally deaf to those cries. To believe, however, that such deafness was peculiarly German, or the result of an aberration in what has otherwise been an inexorable movement towards greater enlightenment, is to feed the very same disease that produced this human catastrophe in the first place. (Lynch 1985: 309)

Since 1948, the World Health Organization has advocated one of the most sophisticated and often quoted definitions of health as 'the state of complete physical, mental and social well-being and not merely the absence of disease and infirmity', which was re-invoked at their conference on New Directions in Health in 1982, when Marsden Wagner bemoaned how medical care used to combine art and technology at a ratio he estimates at 9:1, until medicine became attached to what he describes as 'the rising star of science and classical mechanical physics' (1982: 1207). More recently, at an international Mental Health in Development conference, Professor Norman Sartorius elaborated in painstaking detail how each of the Millennium Development Goals (below) were unachievable without thinking through the mental health implications (Sartorius 2007):

1. Eradicate extreme poverty and hunger
2. Achieve universal primary education
3. Promote gender equality and empower women
4. Reduce child mortality
5. Improve maternal health
6. Combat HIV/AIDS, malaria and other infectious diseases
7. Ensure environmental sustainability
8. Develop a global partnership for development

An enormous challenge lies in the *rapprochement* between social and biological models of health and illness which can, in turn, encompass the political dimensions of the relationship between individuals and the wider social structure. Although we may not be able to find universally valid, comprehensive and agreed definitions of health and illness due to great variability between cultures, historical periods, individuals (and even the same individual over time), instead of remaining embedded in debates between biological and cultural determinism, the way forward surely has to be through an integrated understanding. Whilst biomedical research and scientific progress continue to be vital, it is equally important to advance understanding of the social and socioeconomic factors which play a part in the promotion and maintenance of health and the prevention and causation of disease, and of the relationship between these and the broader social structure.

References

Aakster A (1986) Concepts in alternative medicine. *Social Science and Medicine* 22/2: 265–273.

Abdullah A, Lau Y, Chow L (2003) Patterns of alternative medicine usage among Chinese breast cancer patients: implication for service integration. *American Journal of Chinese Medicine* 31/4: 649–658.

Abraham J (1995) *Science, Politics and the Pharmaceutical Industry: Controversy and Bias in Drug Regulation*. London: Taylor & Francis.

Adams J, Sibbritt DW, Easthope G (2003) The profile of women who consult alternative health practitioners in Australia. *Medical Journal of Australia* 179: 297–300.

American Psychiatric Association (1994) *Diagnostic and Statistical Manual of Mental Disorders*, 4th edn (DSM-IV). Arlington VA: American Psychiatric Association.

Aneshensel CS, Huba GJ (1983) Depression, alcohol use and smoking over one year: a four wave longitudinal causal model. *Journal of Abnormal Psychology* 92/2: 134–150.

Anon. (1993) Complementary therapies in the NHS. Available at www.internethealthlibrary.com/surveys/surveys-uk-comp-therapies-nhs.htm (accessed 27 October 2008).

Antonovsky A (1979) *Health, Stress and Coping*. San Francisco: Jossey-Bass.

Armstrong D (1983) *Political Anatomy of the Body: Medical Knowledge in Britain in the Twentieth Century*. Cambridge: Cambridge University Press.

Armstrong D (1995) The rise of surveillance medicine. *Sociology of Health and Illness* 17/3: 393–404.

Arroba T, James K (1992) *Pressure at Work: A Survival Guide for Managers.* New York: McGraw Hill.

Bauman Z (2000) *Liquid Modernity.* Oxford: Polity Press.

BBC (2006) http://news.bbc.co.uk/go/pr/fr/-/1/hi/health/5007118. stm. See also *HealthWatch* newsletter 62, July 2006 (www. healthwatch-uk.org/newsletterarchive/nlett62.htm).

BBC (2007) www.bbc.co.uk/health.

Beauchamp T, Childress J (1994) *Principles of Biomedical Ethics,* 4th edn. Oxford: Oxford University Press.

Beck U (1992) *Risk Society: Towards a New Modernity.* London: Sage.

Bendelow G (2000) *Pain and Gender.* Harlow: Prentice Hall.

Bendelow G (2006) Pain, suffering and risk. *Health, Risk and Society* 8/1: 1–12.

Bendelow G, Carpenter M, Vautier C, Williams S (eds) (2002) *Gender, Health and Healing: The Public/Private Divide.* London: Routledge.

Bendelow G, Mayall B (2000) How children manage emotion in school. In Fineman S (ed) *Emotion in Organizations,* 2nd edn. London: Sage.

Bendelow G, Williams S (eds) (1998) *Emotions in Social Life.* London: Routledge.

Bernstein BJ, Grasso T (2001) Prevalence of complementary and alternative medicine use in cancer patients. *Oncology* 15: 1267–1272.

Best S (2001) Attention Deficit Disorder: inventing the syndrome to sell the solution. *What Doctors Don't Tell You* 11/11: 1–12.

Black P (2004) *The Beauty Industry: Gender, Culture, Pleasure.* London: Routledge.

Blaxter M (2004) *Health.* Oxford: Polity Press.

Bloom A (ed) (1979) *Toohey's Medicine for Nurses,* 12th edn. London: Churchill Livingstone.

Bolsover N (2002) The 'evidence' is weaker than claimed: Commentary on Holmes J (2002): All you need is cognitive behaviour therapy? Education and Debate Section. *British Medical Journal* 324: 288–294.

Bonica J (1953) *The Management of Pain.* Philadelphia: Lea & Febiger.

Bordo S (1997) *Unbearable Weight: Feminism, Western Culture, and the Body.* Berkeley CA: UCLA Press.

Bordo S, Jagger A (1987) *Gender/Body/Knowledge: Feminist Reconstructions of Being and Knowing.* New Brunswick NJ; London: Rutgers University Press.

Bourdieu P (1984) *Distinction: A Social Critique of the Judgement of Taste*. London: Routledge.

Bower P, Gilbody S (2005) Managing common mental health disorders in primary care: conceptual models and evidence base. *British Medical Journal* 330: 839–842.

Bracken P, Thomas P (2001) Postpsychiatry: a new direction for mental health? *British Medical Journal* 322: 724–727.

Bracken P, Thomas P (2006) *Postpsychiatry: Mental Health in a Postmodern World*. Oxford: Oxford University Press.

Breggin P (2001) *Talking Back to Ritalin: What Doctors Aren't Telling You about Stimulants for Children*. Cambridge MA: Perseus Publishing.

British Medical Association (1993) *Complementary Medicine: New Approaches to Good Practice*. Oxford: Oxford University Press.

British Medical Journal (1997) Editorial. *British Medical Journal* 314: 1594.

Brown G, Harris T (1978) *Social Origins of Depression*. London: Tavistock.

Brown G, Harris T (eds) (1989) *Life Events and Illness*. London: Unwin Hyman.

Bruch H (1978) *The Golden Cage: The Enigma of Anorexia Nervosa*. London: Open Books.

Bury M (1991) The sociology of chronic illness: a review of research and prospects. *Sociology of Health and Illness* 13/4: 451–468.

Busfield J (1996) *Men, Women and Madness: Understanding Gender and Mental Disorder*. London: Macmillan.

Busfield J (ed) (2001) *Rethinking the Sociology of Mental Health*. Sociology of Health and Illness Monograph Series. Oxford: Blackwell.

Cannon WB (1929) *Bodily Changes in Pain, Hunger, Fear and Rage: An Account of Recent Research Into the Function of Emotional Excitement*. New York: Appleton-Century-Crofts.

Cant S, Sharma U (1999) *A New Medical Pluralism? Alternative Medicine and the State*. London: UCL Press.

Cassileth BR (1999) Complementary therapies: overview and state of the art. *Cancer Nursing* 22: 85–90.

Cassileth BR, Schraub S, Robinson E, Vickers A (2001) Alternative medicine use worldwide: the International Union Against Cancer survey. *Cancer* 91: 1390–1393.

Charatan F (2000) US parents sue psychiatrists for promoting Ritalin. *British Medical Journal* 321: 723.

Clarke K (2008) The hardcore gym: culture, practice and knowledge. Unpublished Ph.D. thesis. King's College London.

Cochrane A (1972) *Effectiveness and Efficiency: Random Reflections on the Health Services*. London: Nuffield Provincial Hospital Trust.

Conrad P, Jacobson H (2003) Enhancing biology? Cosmetic surgery and breast augmentation. In Williams S, Bendelow G, Birke L (eds) *Debating Biology: Sociological Reflections on Health, Medicine and Society*, pp 223–34. London: Routledge.

Conrad P, Schneider JW (1992) *Deviance and Medicalization: From Badness to Sickness*. Philadelphia: Temple University Press.

Coward R (1989) *The Whole Truth*. London: Faber & Faber.

Craib I (1994) *The Importance of Disappointment*. London: Routledge.

Datamonitor (2006) survey (www.datamonitor.com).

Department of Health (1991) *The Health of the Nation*. London: HMSO.

Department of Health (1999) *Saving Lives: Our Healthier Nation*. London: HMSO.

Department of Health (2001a) *Mental Health National Service Framework*. London: HMSO.

Department of Health (2001b) *Treatment Choice in Psychological Therapies and Counselling*. London: HMSO.

di Gianni LM, Garber JE, Winer EP (2002) Complementary and alternative medicine use among women with breast cancer. *Journal of Clinical Oncology* 20/18 suppl: 34s–38s.

Dingwall R (1976) *Aspects of Illness*. London: Martin Robertson.

Dobson B (2003) Half of general practices offer patients complementary medicine. *British Medical Journal* 327: 1250.

Dolan A (2007) 'Good luck to them if they can get it': exploring working men's understanding and experiences of income inequality and material standards. *Sociology of Health and Ilness* 29/5: 711–729.

Dubos R (1987) *Mirage of Health: Utopias, Progress, and Biological Change*. New York: Rutgers University Press.

Durkheim E (1897) *Suicide: A Study in Sociology*. London: Routledge & Kegan Paul.

Eisenberg D (1993) Unconventional medicine in the United States. *New England Journal of Medicine* 328: 246–252.

Engel G (1950) Pyschogenic pain and the pain-prone patient. *American Journal of Medicine* 26: 899–909.

Engels F (1987 [1845]) *The Conditions of the Working Class in England*. Harmondsworth: Penguin.

Ernst E (1999) Evidence-based complementary medicine: a contradiction in terms? *Annals of Rheumatism* 58/2: 69–70.

Ernst E (2000) The role of complementary medicine. *British Medical Journal* 321: 119–120.

Ernst E (2006) The 'Smallwood report': method or madness? *British Journal of General Practice* 56/522: 64–65.

Ernst E, Cassileth B (1998) The prevalence of complementary/alternative medicine in cancer: a systematic review. *Cancer* 83: 777–782.

Ernst E, Schmidt K, Steuer-Vogt MK (2003) Mistletoe for cancer? A systematic review of randomised clinical trials. *International Journal of Cancer* 107: 262–267.

Featherstone M (1982) The body in consumer culture. In Featherstone M, Hepworth M, Turner B (eds) *The Body: Social Process and Cultural Theory*. London: Sage.

Fink P, Sørensen L, Engberg M, Holm M, Munk-Jørgensen P (1999) Somatization in primary care: prevalence of health care utilization and General Practitioner recognition. *Psychosomatics* 40/4: 330–338.

Fisher P, Ward A (1994) Medicine in Europe: complementary medicine in Europe. *British Medical Journal* 309: 107–111.

Foucault M (1973) *The Birth of the Clinic*. London: Tavistock.

Fox RC (2002) Medical uncertainty revisited. In Bendelow G, Carpenter M, Vautier C, Williams S (eds) *Gender, Health and Healing: The Public/Private Divide*, pp 236–253. London: Routledge.

Franzen J (2002) *The Corrections*. London: Fourth Estate.

Freund P (1990) The expressive body: a common ground for the sociology of emotions and health and illness. *Sociology of Health and Illness* 12/4: 452–477.

Freund P (1998) Social performances and their discontents. In Bendelow G, Williams S (eds) *Emotions in Social Life*. London: Routledge.

Freund P, McGuire M, Podhurst L (2003) *Health, Illness and the Social Body*, 4th edn. Upper Saddle River NJ: Prentice Hall.

Frey RJ (2007) Stress. In *Encyclopedia of Medicine*. Bnet-United Kingdom. Available at http://findarticles.com/p/articles/mi_g2601/is_/ai_2601001305 (accessed 28 October 2008).

Fulford KWM, Dickenson D, Murray T (2002) *Healthcare Ethics and Human Values*. Oxford: Blackwell.

Furedi F (2004) *Therapy Culture: Cultivating Vulnerability in the Modern Age*. London: Routledge.

Furedi F (2006) Save us from the politics of behaviour. Spiked website 11/11/06.

General Medical Council (1993) *Recommendations on Undergraduate Medical Education*. London: GMC.

General Medical Council (2002) *Tomorrow's Doctors: Recommendations on Undergraduate Medical Education.* London: GMC.

Gislason MK (2007) *Biophilia and Passionate Sociology: Tools for Making Sense of Health, Illness and Disease.* Conference Presentation to the 6th Global Conference on Making Sense of Health, Illness and Disease. University of Oxford. 9–12 July 2007.

Glenton C (2003) Chronic back sufferers: striving for the sick role. *Social Science and Medicine* 57: 2243–2252.

Goffman E (1959) *The Presentation of Self in Everyday Life.* Harmondsworth: Penguin.

Goffman E (1961/1990) *Asylums: Essays on the Social Situation of Mental Patients and Other Inmates.* Harmondsworth: Penguin.

Goldacre B (2007) Spectacularly expensive cost of trial and error. *Guardian* 11 August 2007.

Golding W (1954) *Lord of the Flies.* London: Faber & Faber.

Greco M (2001) Inconspicuous anomalies: alexithymia and ethical relations to the self. *Health* 6/4: 471–492.

Greenhalgh T, Hurwitz B (eds) (1998) *Narrative Based Medicine: Dialogue and Discourse in Clinical Practice.* London: BMJ Books.

Grosz E (1994) *Volatile Bodies: Towards a Corporeal Feminism.* Bloomington/Indianapolis: Indiana University Press.

Hansen E, Easthope G (2006) *Lifestyle in Medicine.* Critical Studies in Health and Medicine. London: Routledge.

Haraway D (1991) *Simians, Cyborgs and Women.* London: Free Association Books.

Health and Safety Executive (HSE) (2008) www.hse.gov.uk/statistics (accessed 11 April 2008).

Healy D (2004) *Let Them Eat Prozac: The Unhealthy Relationship between the Pharmaceutical Industry and Depression.* New York: New York University Press.

Helman C (2007) *Culture, Health and Illness*, 5th edn. Oxford: Arnold/Oxford University Press.

Henderson J, Donatelle R (2004) Complementary and alternative medicine use by women after completion of allopathic treatment for breast cancer. *Alternative Therapies of Health Medicine* 10/1: 52–57.

Hochschild A (1979) Emotion work, feeling rules and social structure. *American Journal of Sociology* 85: 551–575.

Hochschild A (1983, 2003) *The Managed Heart: Commercialization of Human Feeling.* Berkeley CA: University of California Press.

Hochschild A (2005) Rent-a-mom and other services: market, meaning and emotion. *International Journal of Work, Organization and Emotion* 1/1: 74–86.

Hockey J, James A (1993) *Growing Up and Growing Old.* London: Sage.

Holmes J (2002) All you need is cognitive behaviour therapy? Education and Debate Section. *British Medical Journal* 324: 288–294.

Hopper K, Harrison G, Janca A, Sartorius N (2007) *Recovery from Schizophrenia: An International Perspective: A Report from the WHO Collaborative Project, The International Study of Schizophrenia.* Oxford: Oxford University Press.

Hornby N (2001) *How to be Good.* London: Viking.

Huxley A (1932 [1998]) *Brave New World.* New York: Harper Perennials.

Hydén L-C (1997) Ilness and narrative. *Sociology of Health and Illness* 19/1: 48–69.

Illich I (1975) *Limits to Medicine: Medical Nemesis.* London: Calder & Boyars.

James A, Jenks C, Prout A (1998) *Theorizing Childhood.* Cambridge: Polity.

James O (2007) *Affluenza.* London: Vermilion.

Jenkins R (1976) Recent evidence supporting psychologic and social risk factors for coronary disease. *New England Journal of Medicine* 294: 987–994, 1033–1038.

Jewson N (1974) The disappearance of the sick man from medical cosmologies: 1770–1870. *Sociology* 10: 225–244.

Kakai H, Maskarinec G, Shumay D, Tatsumura, Tasaki K (2003) Ethnic differences in choices of health information by cancer patients using complementary and alternative medicine: an exploratory study with correspondence analysis. *Social Science and Medicine* 56/4: 851–862.

Kelly M, Field D (1996) Medical sociology, chronic illness and the body. *Sociology of Health and Illness* 18: 241–257.

Kendell RE (2002) The distinction between personality disorder and mental illness. Review essay. *British Journal of Psychiatry* 180: 110–115.

Kesey, K (1960) *One Flew Over the Cuckoo's Nest.* New York: Picador Books.

Kotarba J (1983) *Chronic Pain: Its Social Dimensions.* Beverly Hills CA: Sage.

Laing RD (1959) *The Divided Self.* London: Tavistock.

Leder D (1984/5) Toward a phenomenology of pain. *Review of Existential Psychiatry* 19: 255–266.

Lewith G, Broomfield J, Prescott P (2002) Complementary cancer care in Southampton: a survey of staff and patients. *Complementary Therapy Medicine* 10/2: 100–106.

Liebling H (2004) Ugandan women's experiences of sexual violence and torture during civil war years in Luwero District: implications for health policy, welfare and human rights. *Psychology of Women Section Review* 6/2: 29–37, autumn edition, BPS.

Liebling-Kalifani H, Marshall A, Ojiambo-Ochieng R, Nassozi M (2007) Experiences of women war-torture survivors in Uganda: implications for health and human rights. *Journal of International Women's Studies* 8/4: 1–17.

Liebling-Kalifani H, Ojiambo-Ochieng R, Marshall A, et al. (2008) Violence against women in Northern Uganda: the neglected health consequences of war. *Journal of International Women's Studies* 9: 4.

Lipowski Z (1988) Somatization: the concept and its clinical application. *American Journal of Psychiatry* 145: 1358–1368.

Lundberg U (2006) Stress, subjective and objective health. *International Journal of Social Welfare* 15/Suppl 1: 41–48.

Lupton D (1995) *The Imperative of Health: Public Health and the Regulated Body*. London: Sage.

Lynch J (1977) *The Broken Heart: The Medical Consequences of Loneliness*. New York: Basic Books.

Lynch J (1985) *The Language of the Heart: The Human Body in Dialogue*. New York: Basic Books.

Lyon M (1996) C. Wright Mills meets Prozac: the relevance of 'social emotion' to the sociology of health and illness. In James V, Gabe J (1996) *Health and the Sociology of Emotions*. Oxford: Blackwell.

Mackenzie E, Taylor L, Bloom B, Hufford D, Johnson J (2003) Ethnic minority use of CAM: a national probability survey of CAM utilizers. *Alternative Therapies in Health and Medicine* Jul–Aug; 9/4: 50–56.

MacLeod U, Ross S, Fallowfield L, Watt GC (2004) Anxiety and support in breast cancer: is this different for affluent and deprived women? *British Journal of Breast Cancer* 91/5: 879–883.

McKeown T (1979) *The Role of Medicine: Dream, Mirage, or Nemesis?* Oxford: Blackwell.

McLaren L, Kuh D (2004) Women's body dissatisfaction, social class, and social mobility. *Social Science & Medicine* 58/9: 1575–1584.

McWhinney I, Epstein R, Freeman T (1997) Rethinking somatization. *Annals of Internal Medicine* 126/9: 747–750.

Malacrida C (2004) Medicalization, ambivalence and social control: mothers' descriptions of educators and ADD/ADHD. *Health* 8/1: 61–80.

Marshall A, Henwood F (2007) Informing health: a participative approach to health information provision. *Library and Information Research* 31/99: 26–40.

Marshall GN, Davis LM, Sherbourne CD (2000) *A Review of the Scientific Literature As It Pertains to Gulf War Illnesses. Volume*

4: *Stress*. Santa Monica CA: Rand Health Communications. www.rand.org.health.

Martin E (1987) *The Woman in the Body*. Milton Keynes: Open University Press.

Martin E (1994) *Flexible Bodies*. Boston MA: Beacon Press.

Martin P, Abraham J, Davis C, Kraft A (2006) Understanding the 'productivity crisis' in the pharmaceutical industry: over-regulation or lack of innovation? In Webster A (ed) *New Technologies in Health Care*, pp 177–193. London: Palgrave.

Marx K (1906–1909) *Capital: A Critique of Political Economy* (3 volumes). Chicago: Charles H. Kerr & Co.

Mayall B (1996) *Children, Health and the Social Order*. Buckingham: Open University Press.

Melzack R, Wall P (1965) Pain mechanisms: a new theory. *Science* 150: 971–979.

Melzack R, Wall P (1988) *The Challenge of Pain*. Harmondsworth: Penguin.

Menkes D (2006) Calling the piper's tune. *Primary Care and Community Psychiatry* 11: 147–149.

Mental Health Act Commission (2007) *Policy Briefing for Commissioners*, issue 17, July. Available at: www.mhac.org.uk/?q=node/12 (accessed 1 November 2007).

Mental Health Foundation (2005) www.mentalhealth.org.uk/ information/mental-health-overview/statistics/.

Mitchell J (1975) *Psychoanalysis and Feminism*. Harmondsworth: Penguin.

Moncrieff J, Hopker S, Thomas P (2005) Psychiatry and the pharmaceutical industry: who pays the piper? *Psychiatric Bulletin* 29: 84–85.

Morris D (1991) *The Culture of Pain*. Berkeley CA; London: University of California Press.

Mullen R, Menkes DB (2008) Psychiatriform disorders: psychiatric analogues of somatoform disorders. *International Journal of Social Psychiatry* 54/5: 395–401.

National Institute for Clinical Excellence (2000) Technology guidance no 13. NICE (www.nice.org.uk).

National Institute for Clinical Excellence (2003) www.nice.org. uk/guidance/t59.

Nettleton S, O'Malley L, Watt I, Duffey P (2004) Enigmatic illness: narratives of patients who live with medically unexplained symptoms. *Social Theory and Health* 2/1: 47–67.

Ni H, Simile C, Hardy AM (2002) Utilization of complementary and alternative medicine by United States adults: results from the 1999 national health interview survey. *Medical Care* 40: 353–358.

Oakley A (1984) *The Captured Womb: A History of the Medical Care of Pregnant Women.* Oxford: Blackwell.

Oakley A (2007) *Fracture: Adventures of a Broken Body.* Bristol: Policy Press.

Orbach S (1986) *Hunger Strike: The Anorectic's Struggle as a Metaphor for our Age.* New York: W. W. Norton & Co.

Parsons T (1951) *The Social System.* Chicago: Free Press.

Petersen A, Bunton R (eds) (1997) *Foucault and Health.* London: Routledge.

Phillips K, Castle D (2001) Body dysmorphic disorder in men. *British Medical Journal* 323: 1015–1016.

Phillips L (2006) *Mental Illness and the Body.* London: Routledge.

Pietroni P (1992) Beyond the boundaries: relationship between general practice and complementary medicine. *British Medical Journal* 305: 564–566.

Pilgrim D (2005) *Key Concepts in Mental Health.* London: Sage.

Porter R (ed) (2002) *The Faber Book of Madness.* London: Faber & Faber

Rees L, Weil A (2001) Editorial: Integrated medicine imbues orthodox medicine with the values of complementary medicine. *British Medical Journal* 322: 119–120.

Reilly D (2001) Comments on complementary and alternative medicine in Europe. *Journal of Alternative and Complementary Medicine* 7/Suppl 1: S23–31.

Reissman CK (1989) Women and medicalization: a new perspective. In Brown P (ed) *Perspectives in Medical Sociology.* Belmont CA: Wadsworth.

Revolutionary Health Committee of Hunan Province (1978) *A Barefoot Doctor's Manual.* London: Routledge & Kegan Paul.

Richardson MA, Sanders T, Palmer JL et al. (2000) Complementary/alternative medicine use in a comprehensive cancer center and the implications for oncology. *Journal of Clinical Oncology* 18: 2505–2514.

Rogers A, Pilgrim D (2005) *A Sociology of Mental Health and Illness*, 3rd edn. Milton Keynes: Open University Press.

Rose H (1994) *Love, Power and Knowledge: Towards a Feminist Transformation of the Sciences.* Cambridge: Polity Press.

Rose N (1998) *Governing the Soul.* London: Routledge.

Ryle G (1949) *The Concept of Mind.* Harmondsworth: Penguin.

Salminen E, Bishop M, Poussa T, Drummond R, Salminen S (2004) Dietary attitudes and changes as well as use of supplements and complementary therapies by Australian and Finnish women following the diagnosis of breast cancer. *European Journal of Clinical Nutrition* 58/1: 137–144.

Samson C (1995) Madness and psychiatry. In Turner B. *Medical Power and Social Knowledge*. London: Sage.

Samson C (1999a) Biomedicine and the body. In Samson C. (ed) *Health Studies: A Critical and Cross-cultural Reader*. Oxford: Blackwell.

Samson C (1999b) Disease and the self. In Samson C. (ed) *Health Studies: A Critical and Cross-cultural Reader*. Oxford: Blackwell.

Saraceno B (2002) Psychiatry's missing diagnosis: social network's healing power is borne out in poorer nations (www.washingtonpost.com/wp-dyn/content/article/2005/06/26/AR).

Sartorius N (2007) *Millennium Development Goals: Risks, Gains and Tasks for Mental Health Programmes*. Plenary, World Psychiatry Association Conference Mental Health in Development, Nairobi, Kenya.

Scambler G (2004) *Health and Social Change: A Critical Theory*. Buckingham: Open University Press.

Scheper-Hughes N, Lock M (1987) The mindful body: a prolegomenon to future work in medical anthropology. *Medical Anthropology Quarterly* 1/1: 6–41.

Schmale A, Iker H (1971) Hopelessness as a predictor of cervical cancer. *Social Science and Medicine* 5: 95–100.

Scott S, Jones D, Cane R, Bendelow G, Fulford KWM (2008) The slide to pragmatism: a values-based understanding of 'dangerous' personality disorders. Wellcome Trust end-of-grant report.

Scull A (1993) *The Most Solitary of Afflictions: Madness and Society in Britain, 1700–1900*. New Haven; London: Yale University Press.

Selye H (1956) *The Stress of Life*. New York: McGraw-Hill.

Shaw M, Dorling D, Gordon D, Davey-Smith G (1999) *The Widening Gap: Health Inequalities and Policy in Britain*. Bristol: Policy Press.

Shilling C (2003 2nd edition) *The Body and Social Theory*. London: Sage.

Showalter E (1987) *The Female Malady: Women, Madness and English Culture 1830–1980*. London: Virago.

Showalter E (1998) *Hystories: Hysterical Epidemics and Modern Culture*. New York: Picador Books.

Siegel B (1989) *Love, Medicine and Miracles*. New York: HarperCollins.

Smallwood C (2005) *The Role of Complementary and Alternative Medicine in the NHS: An Investigation into the Potential Contribution of Mainstream Complementary Therapies to Healthcare in the UK*. London: FreshMinds.

Smith A, Twomey B (2002) Labour market experience of people with disabilities: analysis from the LFS of the characteristics and labour market participation of people with long-term disabilities and health problems. *Labour Market Trends* 110/8: 415–427.

Smith D (1988) *The Everyday World as Problematic*. Milton Keynes: Open University Press.

Smith R (2002) In search of 'non-disease'. *British Medical Journal* 324/7342: 883–885.

Sontag S (1978) *Illness as Metaphor*. New York: Farrar Straus & Giraux.

Strauss A (1975) *Chronic Illness and the Quality of Life*. St Louis: Mosby & Co.

Strong P (1977) Sociological imperialism and the profession of medicine: a critical examination of the thesis of medical imperialism. *Social Science and Medicine* 13A: 199–215.

Summerfield D (2001) The invention of post-traumatic stress disorder and the social usefulness of a psychiatric category. *British Medical Journal* 322: 95–98.

Szasz T (1962) *The Myth of Mental Illness: Foundations of a Theory of Personal Conduct*. New York: Secker & Warburg.

Szasz T (1971) *The Manufacture of Madness*. London: Routledge & Kegan Paul.

Szreter S (1988) The importance of social interaction in Britain's mortality decline 1850–1914: a reinterpretation of the role of public health. *Social History of Medicine*, 1: 1–37.

Tarrier N (2002) Yes, cognitive behaviour therapy may well be all you need: Commentary on Holmes J (2002): All you need is cognitive behaviour therapy? Education and Debate Section. *British Medical Journal* 324: 288–294.

Thoits P (1995) Stress, coping and social support processes: where are we? *Journal of Social Behaviour* (special issue): 53–79.

Tiefer L (2006) Female sexual dysfunction: a case study of disease mongering and activist resistance. *PLoS Medicine* 3/4: e178.

Timimi S (2005) *Naughty Boys: Anti-social Behaviour, ADHD and the Role of Culture*. Basingstoke: Palgrave Macmillan.

Timimi S, Taylor E (2004) ADHD is best understood as a cultural construct. *British Journal of Psychiatry* 184: 8–9.

Tonelli MR (1998) The philosophical limits of evidence based medicine. *Academic Medicine* 73: 1234–1240.

Townsend P, Davidson N (1982) *Inequalities in Health: The Black Report*. Harmondsworth: Penguin.

Tuffs A (2002) Three out of four Germans have used complementary or natural remedies. *British Medical Journal* 325/7371: 990.

Turner B (1996) *The Body and Society*, 2nd edn. London: Sage.

van der Weg W, Streuli R (2003) Use of alternative medicine by patients with cancer in a rural area of Switzerland. *Swiss Medical Weekly* 133/15–16: 233–240.

Wade D, Halligan P (2004) Do biomedical models of illness make for good healthcare systems? *British Medical Journal* 329/7479: 1398.

Wagner M (1982) Getting the health out of people's daily lives. *Lancet* 2/8309: 1207–1208.

Wainwright D, Calnan M (2002) *Work Stress: The Making of a Modern Epidemic*. Buckingham: Open University Press.

Wessely S, Hotopf M, Sharpe M (1998) *Chronic Fatigue and its Syndromes*. Oxford: Oxford University Press.

Whitehead M (1987) *The Health Divide*. London: Health Education Council.

Wilkinson I (2004) *Suffering: A Sociological Introduction*. Cambridge: Polity.

Wilkinson R (1996) *The Impact of Inequality: How to Make Sick Societies Healthier*. London: Routledge.

Williams GH (1984) The genesis of chronic illness: narrative reconstruction. *Sociology of Health and Illness* 6/2: 175–200.

Williams S, Bendelow G (1998) *The Lived Body: Sociological Themes, Embodied Issues*. London: Routledge.

Williams S, Gabe J, Calnan M (eds) (2000) *Health, Medicine and Society: Key Theories, Future Agendas*. London: Routledge.

Winer E (2004) *The Validity of Complementary Therapy Research/ Clinical Trials in Breast Cancer: A Critical Assessment of Where We Are in CAM Research*. Proceedings of 4th European Breast Cancer Conference, Hamburg.

World Health Organization (1992) *The ICD-10 classification of mental and behavioural disorders*. Geneva: World Health Organization.

Wright Mills C (1959) *The Sociological Imagination*. London: Penguin.

Young IM (1990) *Throwing Like a Girl and Other Essays in Feminist Philosophy and Social Theory*. Bloomington: Indiana University Press.

Zaman R, Makhdum A (2000) *Pocketbook of Psychiatry*. London: Churchill Livingstone.

Ziegler F, Imboden JB (1962) Contemporary conversion reactions. II. A conceptual model. *Archives of General Psychiatry* 6: 279–287.

Zola I (1972) Medicine as an institution of social control. *Sociological Review* 20: 487–504.

Websites

BBC health	www.bbc.co.uk/health
Centre for Evidence-Based Medicine, Oxford	www.cebm.net
Datamonitor	www.datamonitor.com
DipEx	www.dipex.org.uk
Emotional health/stress:	www.familydoctor.org
Mental Health Foundation	www.mentalhealth.org.uk
NICE	www.nice.org.uk
Spiked	www.spiked-online.com
WHO and sexology	www.worldsexology.org/

Index

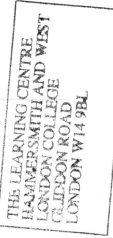

Page numbers in *italics* refer to tables.